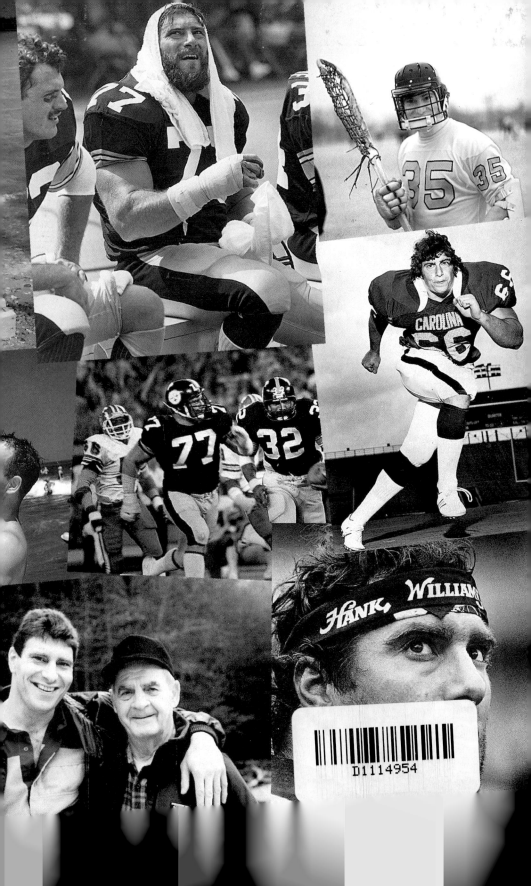

FALSE GLORY

FALSE GLORY

STEELERS AND STEROIDS

The Steve Courson Story

Steve Courson &
Lee R. Schreiber

LONGMEADOW PRESS

-1992-
Happy Valentine's
Day, Brad!
We love you-
Dad & Mom

Published by Longmeadow Press, 201 High Ridge Road, Stamford, CT
06904. All rights reserved. No part of this book may be reproduced or
utilized in any form or by any means, electronic or mechanical, including photocopying, recording or by any information storage and retrieval
system, without permission in writing from the Publisher.

Cover photo © Mike Fabis
Cover design by Mike Stromberg
Interior design by Hannah Lerner
Library of Congress Cataloging-in-Publication Data

ISBN: 0-681-41187-2
Printed in the U.S.

0 9 8 7 6 5 4 3 2 1

To all the athletes
who understand their
limitations

ACKNOWLEDGMENTS

I want to thank the many people who were instrumental in helping the book along to its final end: Tim and Mike Kelley, Dr. August Mauser, Wally Malinchak, Lisa Michalak, Frank Miller, Neil Watko, the Olympia Steele Professional Management Group (especially John Rosenstern and John Lestini), Mike Fabis, Judith and Cathy Malarik, Dr. Jim Wright, my mom, dad and brother, my former teammates (especially Mike Webster, Tunch Ilkin, Craig Wolfley, Gary Dunn, and Ted Petersen) and supporters who provided health care and moral support without which the work on this book would have been impossible. A final special thanks to Chuck Yesalis for his expertise, insight and friendship.

—S.C.

I'd like to thank Daniel Bial, Howard Buck, and Mark Frisk for their professional assistance. And, as always, I'm much obliged to my family for their support and encouragement.

—L.R.S.

CONTENTS

Introduction   1

1 Lost and Found   7

2 Combat and Camaraderie   25

3 Rock and Roll, Sex and Drugs   39

4 Talking Trash and Tactics   61

5 Players and Coaching   81

6 A Tale of Two Cities—Pittsburgh and
  Tampa Bay   99

7 The Article and Its Aftermath   113

8 Hearts and Flowers   129

9 Steroids—An Historical, Medical,
  and Sociological Overview   147

10 Steroids—The Hits and Myths   167

11 Political Football and Fallout   181

12 Present and Future   195

Appendix: Anabolic Steroid Use Among a
          Self-Selected Sample of NFL Players
          *by Charles E. Yesalis, Sc.D.,
          and Stephen P. Courson*   201

INTRODUCTION

I HADN'T SLEPT in five days. My stomach was bloated. I had difficulty breathing. And, try as I might, I couldn't stop those infernal hiccups.

In nine years as a professional football player, I had played with a laundry list of injuries: dislocated foot, dislocated shoulder, hip pointers, pulled hamstrings, sprained ankles, sprained knees, torn knee cartilage. Like many offensive linemen, I also had undergone a couple of knee operations. For most injuries, I took the needle from the team physician, sucked it up, and went out to play.

But this was different from anything I had ever felt before. It wasn't pain, exactly. It was more like disorientation, enervation. Pain I could live with. This was hell.

I knew that I needed medical attention, but I had no health insurance and no funds to cover a lengthy hospital stay. Finally, my friends convinced me to drive to a nearby hospital. The admitting physician said that I looked gray. My blood pressure was 80 over 50. I had absolutely no

1

energy, yet I still couldn't sleep. The doctors refused to give me any sleeping pills, because they wanted me to remain coherent; they hoped my pain would help them figure out what was wrong.

Time passed oh so slowly, painfully so.

I spent eight days in the hospital, the first four in intensive care. I was poked and prodded with various instruments and monitors. An electrocardiogram assessed my heart rate at two hundred beats per minute. They monitored the fluid gathering in my lungs, and then gave me a diuretic to reduce the buildup.

After two days in intensive care, the male nurse who had admitted me stopped by my room. He had worked there for six years, he said, and had never seen anyone who looked as bad as I did make it through the night.

"I expected to read your obit in the paper the next day," he said.

With my regular doctor out of town, a Dr. Rosenbloom took my history. I told him about the football injuries, a background of excessive drinking, and my last anabolic-androgenic steroid (AAS) cycle. Then he sat beside my hospital bed and laid it all out for me: "You have dilated cardiomyopathy, Steve. An enlarged heart in which muscle fibers are lost over time. It's occasionally reversible in the early stages. There are many options we can pursue, the final one being a heart transplant."

I repeated those words in my mind: *Heart. Transplant.*

Prior to that moment, I knew I was pretty sick, but I thought that the worst was behind me. Now I didn't know what to expect.

My entire life had been filled with physical motion, with athletic prowess and achievement. Most of what I had lived for—everything that I had heretofore excelled at—was tied into my physicality. Hitting, blocking, running, jumping, tackling. Lifting, pressing, pushing . . .

Let me get this straight, Doc, those days are over?

"Not necessarily," Dr. Rosenbloom said. "Even heart transplant patients can live relatively active lives." (He didn't mention then that most transplant patients have a life expectancy of five years.)

It was that simple. I was being told that the body that had served me so long and so well had betrayed me. I had just turned 33 years old.

I had just come through some rough times—forced retirement from football, virtual bankruptcy, a battle with alcohol—but this seemed too much, almost beyond my capability.

I knew that once the media got hold of this story it would be distorted: "STEROID ABUSER FACES DEATH . . ." "HEART TRANSPLANT NEEDED BY AVID ABUSER STEVE COURSON . . ."

All the things I had accomplished—a Pro Bowl alternate with two Super Bowl rings; an integral part of perhaps the most successful football team ever; and then a world-class powerlifter—would be reduced to a footnote. I was the guy who had blown the whistle on rampant steroid use in the NFL, who had volunteered this information, mind you, without being caught, and who had accused coaches and league officials of ignoring the problem at best; at worst, of encouraging it. I had already been perceived by some as a zealot, a bitter and monomaniacal behemoth who couldn't get off his soapbox.

And now I was "that steroid guy" who needed a new heart.

What exactly caused my condition is open to argument. Perhaps I had a bad batch of genes. I was adopted at 10 months and never knew my biological mother and father. Alcoholism is often linked with cardiomyopathy, and Lord knows, I've done my fair share of drinking.

When you ask my doctors whether steroids brought me to this pass, they say they were "contributing factors." If I had never taken steroids, or taken fewer of them, quite possibly the disease would not be as bad, or it would have taken longer to develop. Who knows? Research is spotty, at best. The doctors point out that had my heart wall been thick instead of thin, my illness could have been linked more directly to AAS usage. But if I had never taken steroids, I probably would have drunk less too. No doubt about it, steroid use leads to all sorts of changes in personality and behavior as well as in your physical self. I—and many others—became aggressive, highly sexed, primed for anything when I was cycling steroids. I felt invulnerable.

Lying in a hospital bed, being told my life was virtually over, changed all that. It's too late for me to cry over decisions I've made. I loved the strength and the body steroids helped give me. I loved playing football for the Pittsburgh Steelers. But what is important now is for me to focus on getting better, and to utilize whatever time I have left in the most productive way possible.

At this writing, it's been nearly three years since I was diagnosed with dilated cardiomyopathy, and I still have the same ineffectual organ ticking inside. Without a transplant, they say, a person in my condition should survive anywhere from three to five years. That means I'm past halftime, well into the third quarter.

Like many people in my situation, I've tried to use my illness for some good. I've made it the focal point of my crusade against the ignorance surrounding steroids and other prevalent ills in organized sports. It's the hook that often gets people to listen: "Heart transplant candidate speaks out on steroid use." If that's what gets them in the tent, I can live with that. (And all this time, I thought it was my good looks.)

In order to speak credibly, I have researched the steroid issue like no other layperson. I have given talks at medical conventions, schools, and colleges. Kids respond to me because they know I won't lie to them. Nor will I use scare tactics to try and frighten them.

This crusade, my mission, is a compulsion to tell the truth: about the use and abuse of steroids, as well as other illegal and legal drugs; about the corruption and venality in organized sports; about the multitude of abuses in college and pro sports; and about what I perceive to be a conspiracy of silence by all these powers-that-be in order to maintain the status quo (and protect their collective rears). I will tell the truth as I know it for as long as I can, and for as long as people will listen.

So far, the doctors say that my condition has "stabilized." Because of my size—I'm now 6'1" and 280 pounds (in my playing days, I was up to 295)—I am going to need an unusual donor, one whose heart is large enough for my frame. At some point in the near future, in order to move up on the transplant list, I will have to check myself into the hospital.

Believe it or not, some folks out there have said that I should not even be eligible for a transplant, that as a drug abuser I should not take a "good, clean person's" spot. Fortunately, the doctors don't share that view.

Most of my life I have worked, trained, and fought to prove something to myself and others. As a student of military history, I knew that the best-prepared and-conditioned soldiers survive. But I was never quite sure who I was fighting against, or what I was really trying to prove. Was it a desire to be *somebody*? Was it fueled by a need to achieve? Or was it in some way compensation for being abandoned at birth?

Again, the precise reasons don't seem to matter much now.

For most of my life, I have been a man of action; introspection is difficult, often painful. But with nothing left to prove, I am finally free to find out who the hell I am, and—if given half the chance—who I am going to become.

1

LOST AND FOUND

I WAS ABANDONED at birth by a 19-year-old girl. I use the word
"abandoned" for effect; I have no idea what went through
my mother's mind when she put me up for adoption
immediately after my birth on October 1, 1955. All I know
about my biological mother was that she came from a
Philadelphia family of lawyers and was of Swedish descent.
I do not know anything about my biological father.

At the age of 10 months, I was adopted by Iber and
Elizabeth Courson, God-fearing Lutherans from Glenside,
Pennsylvania. My father worked as an engineer, and my
mother as a nurse. My older brother, Bruce, was adopted six
years earlier under similar circumstances.

Uncharacteristically, I have not tried to trace my background. Nor have I asked many questions concerning my
lineage. Only recently, since my heart illness, have I given
it some real thought: I've wondered if there could be a
genetic link to my cardiomyopathy. The adoption agency

originally told my parents that there was no history of serious disease in my background.

When I was younger, my parents gave me numbers I could call if I was inclined to look into it further; they certainly never discouraged me. But I suppose that I've never really cared enough to pursue it primarily because I thought it might hurt them. My adoptive parents are my parents. Even now, when I go back to Gettysburg to visit them, I feel as if I'm home, although I've basically been on my own since I was 17. When I left the hospital in the fall of 1988, after being diagnosed with the heart disease, I was in need of some tender loving care, so I went to stay with my parents for a time. I came home.

My parents are not particularly demonstrative people— they've never been comfortable with public displays of affection—but I've always felt loved and supported.

I, too, have some difficulty expressing overt affection and emotion. In that way, I am my parents' child. Yet, as I've come to realize the transience and importance of each moment, I've tried to let my mom and dad know how much I appreciate what they've done for me over the years, and how much I do love them.

Even now, it's probably easier for me to express these feelings on paper than to speak directly to them. But I'm working on it.

As a kid growing up in Longmeadow, Massachusetts, I was pretty typical: quiet, liked to read, a good student and a Boy Scout. My parents wanted me to be well rounded, so I took up the string bass. I was already a little big for my age, and that seemed like a suitably sized instrument. For some reason, I was fascinated with the military; early on, I had aspirations of going to West Point. My favorite television show was "Combat," with Vic Morrow.

Though my parents never pushed me into sports, I

excelled at them. One of my earliest memories, at around four, was having a catch with my father. I remember making a bad throw, and my father was unable to move and catch it. He had badly damaged knees from playing high school and college football and could not be as active as other fathers his age.

We had a lot of kids in the neighborhood—this was a typical suburban setting in the early sixties—and we played sandlot everything: baseball, basketball, softball, kickball. The other boys were not too thrilled about playing football with me; apparently I played a little too "physically" for them.

At age 11, I went out for pee-wee football and broke my thumb during preseason drills. I told my football coach that I couldn't play in the first game because my thumb was broken (and also that my parents had tickets to a big Red Sox game during the '67 pennant drive), and he began yelling at me in front of all the kids. I went home crying.

That incident, and that insensitive coach, so traumatized me that I didn't play football again for three years.

In ninth grade I decided that I wanted to play football again. My dad worried that I'd be prone to quitting. In his day, the late 1930s, he went about 5'10", 205 pounds—and from what I hear he was a pretty fair offensive tackle. He just wanted me to be as serious about the game as he had been.

My mother, who was not a big sports fan—and not a fan at all of football—refused at first to sign the permission slip.

"But Mo-o-m!" I whined and wailed and pleaded.

Who could resist such a compelling argument? She signed the slip, and my career in football was set.

The following year, as a sophomore at Longmeadow High School (the third-ranked academic school in Massachusetts), I was a varsity starter, playing both sides of the line of scrimmage. This was about the time I began weightlifting—which was not, back in 1970, the most popular endeavor, athletically or socially. In addition to lettering in football, I also played varsity lacrosse and baseball. As an honor student, my best subjects were history, science, and social studies.

Right before my senior year, because of my father's business, we moved to Gettysburg, Pennsylvania,—site of the renowned Civil War battle—where football was king.

Gettysburg High was much easier for me academically—I barely cracked the spine of a book and still made all A's and B's—while the level of football play was much tougher. I like to think that I rose to the competitive challenge. While anchoring the offensive and defensive lines, and even playing some linebacker, I made All-Conference both ways and was named a Harrisburg-area Blue Chipper—an honor that usually garnered some serious interest from the top college scouts.

Historically, Pennsylvania has had an inordinate number of successful athletes—particularly football players—come out of its steel towns and mining country. Guys like Mike Ditka, who played at Aliquippa High School; Joe Namath, from Beaver Falls; George Blanda, Youngwood; Tony Dorsett, Hopewell High; Joe Montana, Ringold High; and Dan Marino, Central Catholic High School. There are many, many more.

The likely reason is that our parents were hard-working people with strong values. Nothing was ever given to us, so, early on, we had to take some control of our lives. Certainly, the shot-and-a-beer mentality—work hard, play hard—might've rubbed off on a few of us good ol' boys.

I was also fortunate that my high school football coach, Leo Ward, was one of the good ones. Leo liked to work out with his team. And because he didn't ask us to do anything that he wouldn't do, we respected him. He also seemed to respect us. Sure, he might ream us out for a bonehead play.

But by and large, he treated us like young men—not boys, not fools, not dogs. Many of my subsequent mentors could've learned a thing or three from Leo.

Under Leo's guidance, I stepped up my weight training; I even supplemented it by taking protein tablets. One time, in psychology class, the pills fell out of my pocket and the teacher saw them. She accused me of having a drug problem, which I denied. In fact, drugs were prevalent in the school, and most of my friends smoked pot. But at that time the only drug I took was aspirin.

As a result of my training, I was eventually able to bench-press 400 pounds; I could also dunk a basketball and run 4.7 in the 40-yard dash. Although I had the grades and SATs to get into an Ivy League school, I decided that I wanted a taste of big-time college football. Interest was shown by Kansas State, Colorado, Penn State, and South Carolina, as well as smaller schools—such as Bucknell, Penn, and Delaware—where education was more emphasized.

After talking it over at length with my parents, I signed a grant-in-aid to the University of South Carolina. I liked their pitch; they saw me as a big, fast linebacker—a vision I shared. The coaches anticipated, as did I, that with my size and speed I could dominate the position.

I reported to summer practice in Columbia, South Carolina, in the beastly hot August of 1973. It would not be unusual for the temperature on the turf to reach 120 degrees Fahrenheit. Nor would it be unusual for us to practice three times a day in this heat.

The whole environment was a distant cry from the high spirits and high jinks of high school football. Bigger people, bigger pressure, bigger business. And let me tell you: This was *serious* business.

The coaches, under the leadership of head coach Paul Dietzel (formerly of West Point, often called "Pepsodent

Paul" because of his winning smile), were under great pressure from the media, the fans, and the administration, which was no doubt under great pressure from the boosters and alumni. And all this pressure came down squarely on the tightly cropped heads of 18-, 19-, 20-, 21-, and 22-year-old young men. I was, at 17, the youngest of them.

The hazing process of the S.C. freshmen began quite early. For me and my rookie mates, it started with our first team meal. We were blithely chowing down at the Roost— the athletic dorm complex dubbed for our school nickname, the Fighting Gamecocks—when the veteran players convened the hazing session. Each of us new kids was required to get on a table in the middle of the cafeteria and bark out like Marinesin response to several basic questions.

I was one of the first to stand up and do my spiel— orchestrated, of course, to a full chorus of boos. A number of other freshmen followed me to the podium, with the same results. Then a rather stocky lineman type, wearing bib overalls and sporting a crew cut—this kid had country written all over him—got up and began to reveal his résumé.

Name? "Mike Wood."

High school? "Elizabethton, Tennessee."

Position? "Defensive tackle."

Honors?

Mike was stumped; perhaps he hadn't received any honors back in Elizabethon. Finally, he puffed up his big chest and blurted: "Well, I'm jes honored to be here!"

The place just shook with laughter. The hazing was over. We were a team.

With the coaches breaking the team down into several subgroups, I worked out with the linebackers and tight ends. Although I was, at 230, the heaviest player in the group, I finished second in the mile run. The coaches were impressed. Along with just a few other freshmen, I was immediately elevated to the varsity. And because South Carolina needed some help on the defensive line, I was moved right in there—alternating at tackle with a senior.

Practices were brutal. This was my first taste of Astro-Turf, and it wasn't a pleasant one—not with temperatures hovering around triple digits every day; the artificial surface sucked up every degree of the heat and humidity. It was also my initiation into the world of assistant coaches, intransigent Southern ones to boot. And I learned a new definition of the term "loaf."

To these assistant coaches, many of whom had grown up in these hot, humid parts, anything less than full-out effort at all times was considered a "loaf." For those of us on the defensive line, a loaf was something less than complete pursuit of the ball until the whistle was blown. If a player stopped because he thought the play was dead, we'd hear: "Would your mama be proud of that loaf, boy?" Or: "Son, you aren't loafin', are ya?"

Of course, the mere fact that the question was asked meant that we *were* loafing. The punishment for a loaf was five sprints, 40 yards apiece. If you were unfortunate enough to rack up three loafs per practice, you'd be tacking on 15 40-yard sprints to the 20 40-yard sprints that normally ended each practice.

Our morning and afternoon practices were a minimum of two hours in full pads. For evening sessions, which lasted nearly as long, we were permitted to wear shorts. One morning, after a full round of sprints in 9,000-degree weather, I collapsed and was hospitalized for heat prostration. The next day, I was greeted with the usual sullen grunts and expected to return to full practice—to the sprints, the drills, the scrimmaging, and the stench.

Oh, yes, I neglected to mention the indescribably foul

odor that filled the stagnant air during morning practice. Our field was near an old meat-packing plant, and mornings were apparently the best time to burn the plant's waste products. What a wonderful way to start the day.

Because college football seemed to me so unbelievably grueling, there were many times that I thought about quitting. That or punching one of them redneck assistant coaches. But the even more dismal prospect of losing my scholarship and dropping out of school to join the real world probably kept me from doing anything too rash.

In truth, I was committed to football. While I had certain doubts and complaints about the coaching methods, I rarely expressed them. I was prepared to do whatever it took to get the job done. And, frankly, that's all the coaches were concerned about: Could I do the job? Was I man enough to get it done?

Most coaches don't much care if a player is overmatched and outmanned. They're not interested in your fears, doubts, the fact that you might be playing a new position. It doesn't matter if you're a rookie or a veteran. Only one key question: Can you do the job?

And so, if the coaches wanted me to run sprints, I sprinted. If they wanted me to run drills, I drilled. And if they wanted me to play defensive tackle, I'd tackle anyone they put in front of me.

The first game of the season, our home opener against Georgia Tech, was played at night in front of more than 50,000 screaming fans. I knew I wasn't in Gettysburg anymore, where a few thousand rabid rooters cheered for the hometown high school heroes. This was different. This was electric. This was big-time NCAA ball.

Playing against older, more experienced players, I felt almost like a boy among men, particularly at my new position. In the second game of my college career, I, a 6'1",

230-pound, 17-year-old freshman defensive tackle, was matched against Houston's all-conference guard, Everett Little. Everett was three or four years older and went 6'5", 285 pounds. I was overmatched and outmanned indeed; but I was also young, cocky, and probably a little naïve. I didn't know enough to be scared. I only wanted to show the coaches that they had made the right choice, that I could do the job. And I suppose that, other than the beating Little gave me that day, I did my job well enough on the field that season.

In the meantime, there were a couple of other adjustment problems that I was experiencing at South Carolina. There was, for example, that old-time religion.

I had been raised up North as a devout Lutheran. I believed in the Golden Rule and the separation of church and state. But down here, there didn't seem to be much separation between church and/or state and/or football.

Before our biggest game of the season—against our most hated rival, the Clemson Tigers (over the years, the National Guard had occasionally been called in to quell disturbances at these matchups)—we received a most unusual pep talk from our team chaplain, minister of the largest Baptist congregation in Columbia. He spoke passionately on the importance of winning, of doing our best, and of crushing the Tigers' spirits and bodies.

Then, in a graphic, almost frenzied demonstration, he poured a box of plucked chicken feathers onto the meeting-room floor.

"Men," he said with unadulterated solemnity, "this is what those Clemson boys think of the Fighting Game-cocks!"

This little demonstration confused me, theologically and philosophically. Why should God care whether S.C. beat Clemson?

For a long time thereafter, I questioned the teachings of the church and how it could allow its tenets to be subverted with this win-at-all-cost mentality. Sports, it seemed to me then, had been elevated into some newfangled fundamentalist religion. And even as a pious young parishioner in the church of Football, it seemed to me a serious breach of priorities. I did not understand then, and I still don't understand, why athletes and coaches feel compelled to compete for Christ (or Allah). I don't recall the Bible mentioning anything about winning and losing. I decided then that I'd play, but I wouldn't pray.

Most of us Gamecocks were glad to see the season end. We had a relatively successful campaign at seven and four, but the torrid pace and pressure had burned most of us out. We were so eager to take a break from the game that we rooted—literally—against going to a bowl. If Georgia Tech were to beat Georgia in their final game, we'd be getting a bid to the Peach Bowl. Many of us gathered—seniors included—cheering for the Bulldogs to beat Tech. Fortunately for us, they did. I'm sure the coaches, the boosters, and administration weren't too thrilled with the lost revenues, but most of the players were positively giddy.

In terms of extracurricular revenue for students—such as illegal payments or no-show jobs—South Carolina was not, at least in my day, a major violator. The transgressions, such as there were, seemed pretty limited. Essentially, players subsisted on scalping Clemson tickets (we could usually get about $25 for each ticket) and cashing laundry checks ($15 per month.) More substantial payments may have been slipped to some players under the table, but I never received any, nor did any of my friends. I don't even recall seeing a teammate ride around in a fancy car. Other than our scholarships, we were essentially slave labor.

Slave labor fueled, in some cases, by artificial means.

While training during the summer of '74, before my sophomore year, it dawned on me that once again I'd be facing offensive linemen who topped out at 270, 280. I thought it might be wise if I tried to put on a few pounds of my own, get some gristle on that bone.

That summer I stayed down in Columbia, living off campus and training at the school's athletic facilities. One day, I remember working out in the weight room with one of the assistant coaches, a guy whom I liked and respected because he trained as hard as his players. We were both doing some bench presses, and I noticed there were some little blue pills in a bowl on a nearby table. The coach, half kiddingly, said to me: "Hey, Steverino, maybe you should try some of these."

The pills were Dianabol, the first American steroid. They were sitting in a corner, available to anyone who stuck his hands in the bowl.

I went to one of the team physicians and told him that I wanted to gain weight. I asked him, "What about steroids?" I first heard of them when I was about 12; a friend's sister was dating a football player from Texas, and this guy had bulked up big time using steroids. I didn't observe any firsthand usage in high school; but, at college, other players had often suggested that I take them.

This team doctor asked no questions. He simply took my blood pressure and handed me a prescription for 30 five-milligram tablets of Dianabol, the same pills I had seen in the weight room. He said to take in a lot of protein. I took the prescription to the local pharmacy, and the university was billed—again, no questions asked.

When I opened up my first bottle of Dianabol, I read the attached insert: "These drugs do not enhance athletic ability." Well, I thought, we'd find out soon enough.

I took one tablet a day for 30 days. I ate like a pig and trained like a maniac. One month later, my weight went from 232 to 260 pounds, my dashes were the fastest times of my life (as low as 4.5), while my bench presses went up 50 pounds (to about 450). That's *fifty*—five-oh!—pounds in 30 days.

Gee, I wonder if they had enhanced my athletic ability in any way. Who the hell are they kidding?!!

During this time, I also played basketball, ran, and lifted weights five days a week, while eating at least one pound of red meat, chicken, or fish per day—in addition to stuffing my face with any other morsels I found in my path.

I couldn't believe how productive I had become in my training. It was actually an incentive to put in *more* time in the gym, and I soon became a fanatic. That's why when I hear talk of "cheating," it's really a misnomer. And it pisses me off mightily. Guys on steroids usually work twice as hard; they're not looking for a quick fix. They're among the most motivated athletes in the world, and they're willing to do whatever it takes to get the job done—side effects or long-term damage be damned.

When I reported to training camp in the late summer, the coaches were pleased. No one said anything to me specifically, but they certainly noticed my increased bulk, strength, and speed.

From that time on, I was a chemically augmented athlete. For every major athletic event in which I was to participate for the rest of my life, I no longer relied on natural adrenaline or even processed sugar to pump me up. I was artificially pumped—and pleased. My coaches were happy. The only person who was not real thrilled was my mom.

When I came home for a short break before school started, my mother took one look at me and said, "What the heck is going on?" I told her what drug I had taken, and who had prescribed it for me. My mother the nurse got out her little book on pharmacology and made me read all about the potential side effects. She even pointed out the literature that read, "These drugs don't enhance athletic ability."

Sure, Mom, I've seen all that stuff already. Then who was this 260-pound man mountain in your kitchen who could run a 4.5 forty and bench press more than 450? I was obviously not the same fellow who had left home a few months earlier. But that was 1974, back in the dark ages, and this stuff was so deep in the closet that no one was talking about it. And no one knew a damn thing about it.

I explained to her that a school doctor had okayed the drugs—the university was even paying for them—so how bad could they be? (Later, I went to a local physician, and he prescribed 2.5 milligrams of Dianabol—half the dosage I had been taking. He, too, had no idea what he was giving me.)

I also tried to tell my mother that college football was a business, and I needed to take these prescribed "enhancers" in order to keep my job. But being a very conservative, middle-class, middle-aged woman—and a concerned parent—my mother did not like me taking drugs of any kind.

Back in training camp, I found a slight downside to the Dianabol. Because of all the added bulk, my tendons were under increased strain; I soon developed tendonitis, particularly in my shoulders. And within several weeks I experienced my first severe football injury—a freak incident precipitated by poor body position—which would be the first of many knee injuries. It happened on an inside hamburger drill—offensive line squaring off against defensive line—and I had never felt such pain. The diagnosis was a strained medial collateral ligament in my right knee, which would likely require four to six weeks of rest and rehabilitation.

During that time, the team did poorly; we got ripped by Georgia Tech, Duke, and then Georgia. The day after the Georgia game, on a Sunday while the team was still banged up, we were forced to practice on the steaming carpet of Williams Brice Stadium. Even thought I was hurt, I was forced to attend. And, just in case people couldn't identify the injured players, we were all outfitted in white jerseys with a big red cross on them. The insensitivity of these coaches was amazing. I never forgot nor have I ever forgiven them for that humiliating little stunt.

Before I could even scrimmage with the team, the Fighting Gamecocks were 0-5 and the fans, administration, and alumni were screaming for the head of Coach Dietzel (who would be gone after that season). Though he was obviously feeling the heat, Dietzel was still pitching that salesman's smile and trying to inspire us with his motivational speeches. I remember the one before the North Carolina game, in which he told us that we should play for our own pride, and not for the coaches, and that our very manhood was under scrutiny. One of the last things he said before we ran out onto the field was particularly memorable. He told us to "go out there and knock the pee out of them!" That was his very word: pee.

We were trying so hard not to laugh that a few of us may have knocked a little pee out of ourselves.

During my rehabilitation, one positive thing did occur: I was switched to the offensive line, a position I found most naturally suited to my talents and personality. The downside was that one of our senior captains, Jerry Witherspoon, was playing ahead of me. The last game of the season, against our archrival Clemson, Jerry went down early with an ankle injury, and I got to play the rest of the game at guard.

We eventually lost in a close one to a fine Clemson team,

but I felt as if I had found my true position. I was bursting out on run blocks with ruthless efficiency, utilizing my added size and strength to thoroughly neutralize opposing linemen and backers. I'm not normally given to overly sentimental thoughts, but that day was one of *those* days: perfect football weather, crisp and sunny; a screaming crowd; a feeling of mastery at my job. I remember thinking: *This is it; this is where I should be.* No doubt, part of the euphoria was simply being young, having my entire life ahead of me and feeling that I could accomplish anything.

By the time I was a senior, I had become a very accomplished offensive guard and was attracting some attention from pro scouts. At a combined scouting workout, on a rainy day with a slight hamstring pull, I was clocked in 4.8 for the 40-yard dash—not my best time, but very credible considering the conditions.

I couldn't wait for college to be over. While many of my friends were wondering what to do with their lives, I knew that I'd be playing professional football or die trying.

My college football career ended on the losing end of a poorly played game in Death Valley, home of the Clemson Tigers. The day was appropriately gray and drizzly, and it seemed like we had saved all of our season's turnovers for that final game.

At the end of the season, South Carolina printed a program of the Fighting Gamecocks' football team with all of the seniors on the cover. Out of 70 scholarship athletes who had begun the S.C. football program four years prior, only 13 seniors remained. I felt like I had come through a particularly protracted and grueling Marine boot camp, with most of the grunts having washed out.

It's a wonder that any of us made it. I thought of all the times that I or my teammates had gone down with heat prostration and had to be carried off the field packed in ice. I thought of the "barf buckets," kept on the sidelines during the extraordinarily brutal winter workouts, and how if a player used them, he was ridiculed mercilessly by the coaches as a "weakling." And I could recall friends of mine getting their knees blown out, writhing in pain on the turf, while the coaches pushed through the huddle around the injured player and hollered, "Get another body in here."

I wondered if it would be any different in the pros.

The post-college season soon began in earnest. I was named to the All-South Independent team and played in the Blue-Gray Game, as well as the East-West Shrine Game. I played well in both contests and anticipated possibly moving up into one of the early rounds of the pro draft.

Then all I could do was wait. I waited alone in my room for the phone call that would change my life. Where would I be spending the next several years? Would I be going to a rock-solid franchise or a rebuilding program? Could I crack the starting lineup? How much money would I be making?

I had considerable time to ask myself every imaginable question as the day dragged on without a call—through the morning and afternoon, and then into the evening. I went to dinner thinking the worst: I might not be picked by any team.

About 9 P.M. I received a call from Dick Haley, director of player personnel for the Pittsburgh Steelers, informing me that I had been selected as the second of the team's three fifth-round draft picks. Being from the Gettysburg area, several dozen miles southeast of Pittsburgh, I was ecstatic.

I left my room to get some fresh air and immediately ran into a friend of mine from Pennsylvania who'd come by to check on my draft status. When I told him that I'd soon be heading for the Steelers' training camp, he whooped joyfully and then tackled me. We continued to celebrate pretty strenuously that night.

In the next couple of days it began to sink in: I was going

to get a shot with the Pittsburgh Steelers. Over the previous three years, the Steelers had won two Super Bowls and almost made it into a third, losing in the AFC championship game to the Raiders, the eventual NFL champions. I wondered what I could offer a team so successful and storied.

I wondered if I could do the job.

2

COMBAT AND CAMARADERIE

RIGHT BEFORE MY rookie season with the Steelers in 1977, I took three 5-milligram tablets of Dianabol a day for six weeks. Compared to present-day dosages, 15 milligrams was like taking extra-strength aspirin. Yet this was still three times greater than any cycle I had done in college, where I had never ingested more than one of those robin's-egg-blue pills in a single day.

My main motivation for using the drug was simple: I was about to enter the training camp of the world-champion Pittsburgh Steelers, and I was expected to block All-Pros such as Joe Greene and Ernie Holmes to make the team. That's the predominant reason why most athletes use these performance-enhancing drugs—to compete at a higher level, and to compete evenly with their opponents. I don't believe Joe or Ernie used steroids—in those days, few defensive linemen did—but several of my rivals on the offensive line certainly did.

My intention was to succeed at this game, no matter

25

what the cost. Ironically, in those days the medical world was still claiming "placebo," maintaining that these drugs didn't really work. Anyone who used them knew what a load of shinola that was. It was evident to me—and to anyone who observed me over a month's time—that these things worked remarkably well. Nor did I see any damaging health effects in myself or my peers. Perhaps if guys were dropping like flies in practice, I might have rethought my position. But back then there seemed to be only enormous benefits and few, if any, drawbacks.

Steeler training camp was (and still is) at St. Vincent College in Latrobe, PA home of Arnold Palmer and Rolling Rock beer. Avid fans would often plan their vacations around these eight grueling weeks of boot camp and on any given day there might be as many as ten thousand spectators watching us work.

Since I was a fifth-round draft choice (technically 5b), the Steelers were expecting just some lineman/linebacker from a middling program. Instead, I strode into camp a marbled 265 and ran the 40 in 4.6 seconds; I was also bench pressing in the upper 400s, which immediately made me one of the strongest guys on the team.

Though thoroughly juiced and pumped, I was not a happy camper. After several weeks, I was still having difficulty adapting to the Steelers' offensive system. It wasn't physical or mental inferiority; it was mainly the adjustment to the pro game.

At that time, college offensive linemen couldn't use their hands to block—though the pros were allowed to—so I had to unlearn old techniques and learn completely new ones. I could see why offensive linemen needed so much upper-body strength and bulk; pro blocking was all about gaining leverage with arms and hands. And it became equally apparent why it was necessary to use some artificial enhancement to help get that edge.

Over the years the college rules have been changed, mainly to protect quarterbacks, and the transition for an offensive lineman into the pros is no longer that great. But back then, in training camp I felt like I was playing with at least one hand tied behind my back, while the biggest, strongest athletes on the planet were teeing off on me with impunity.

Actually it was no shame to have my butt kicked by the likes of Joe Greene, L. C. Greenwood, and Ernie Holmes. These guys were Super Bowl champs and one of the greatest defensive lines of all time—the fabled Steel Curtain.

After exhibition season, Steelers' head coach Chuck Noll came up to me and said: "Steve, we think you have potential to play here, but you're not going to make the team. You have a choice: We can waive you and you can try to hook on with another team, or we can put you on injured reserve." Of course, I was not hurt—though they announced to the league that I had an "ankle injury." In subsequent years, the NFL began cracking down on that practice of falsely protecting players.

I told Chuck that I wanted to play with the Steelers, so I agreed to stay, even if it meant that I wasn't really part of the team. Or at least that's how it felt to me. My job was to simply help with the "offensive picture"—simulating the blocking schemes as close to game conditions as possible. I may have been a sub-Steeler, but I was facing off against bona fide Steelers.

That first year was a clinic. It taught me how to swallow dirt and keep my mouth shut. I learned what to do with my hands, and how to get the most leverage. Mostly I watched the games on TV like any other fan. The Steelers finished the 1977 season with 9–5 record and then lost to Denver in the first round of the playoffs. I definitely felt that I could have helped the team.

During the off-season I trained like a maniac. I knew that

I'd again be fighting for a job. But I also knew that I could hold my own against anyone on the Steelers, or in the league.

In an early 1978 exhibition game against the Cowboys, I was matched up against All-Pro defensive end Randy White. The previous preseason he had wiped my rear all over the turf. This time, on the first play of the game, I fired out on a run block and flattened him ass over teakettle. He might not have been as motivated as I—at least at the start—but he got real serious real fast. Even so, I played him even up for the rest of that afternoon.

In practice, I usually lined up across from Ernie Holmes on straight-ahead run-blocking drills. Ernie's reputation around the league was as one of the most fearsome defensive linemen against the run; he was particularly devastating on the one-on-one block, since it usually took more than one man to route him out of there.

For an entire year, Ernie had dominated me—pushing and smacking me around at will. Ernie was a ferocious game-player, and—when he wanted to be—just as fierce in practice. I practiced hard, but I rarely looked to hurt the guy across from me.

It seemed so unnecessary and even childish to go after your teammates with such a vengeance. Yet the coaches seemed to foster this attitude. It was as if they felt a player wouldn't know the difference between practice and a game. Nor could I ever figure out why coaches would almost encourage us to fight with each other in practice. Supposedly it showed them that we had the fire and abandon to hurt our opponents on Sunday.

I preferred to bank my fires until game time, when it counted. Of course, Chuck Noll, like most NFL coaches, felt somewhat differently, and even up until my last days with the Steelers six years later, he was still reaming me out about my lackadaisical practice habits.

"You practice like you play!" Chuck used to scream at us. Well, if the Steelers of that era really practiced like we played, none of us would've made it through a season.

Anyway, on this day in practice, I was fired up. I wanted to prove to Chuck Noll and my teammates that I wasn't just some scrubeenie kept around for teeing-off practice. On the first drill, I came off the ball with perfect technique, driving Ernie back six or eight yards and eventually knocking him down. Like most folks who earn their living at football, Ernie had a bit of a temper. (A couple of years before, Ernie had been arrested for shooting out truck tires with a rifle on the Ohio Turnpike.) But this was the first time that I had ever stuck it to him in this drill. And boy, was he pissed.

We lined up again, and though it was a relatively warm day in Pittsburgh, I swore I could see steam coming out of from Ernie's mask. Again, it was the same result: I dusted his ass. I thought for sure he was going to punch me out.

Right about then, there was a buzz around the practice field: the kid's whipping Ernie's big butt. It was like a bad TV movie. Was this the pivotal moment in the story when the youngster finally earns the grizzled veteran's grudging respect? Or was this the moment that the kid gets to swallow his teeth?

In real life, of course, nobody got his bridgework bashed. And nobody patted my rear in approval. Certainly Ernie was still too steamed at the time to say anything; I think he would've liked to simply stomp on my face. But from that moment on, the coaches and the other players did treat me differently. That is, they treated me the same as anyone else on the team.

I was a Steeler.

Facing off against other Steelers—including the great "Mean" Joe Greene—usually meant a different sort of confrontation. Joe was no less fierce a competitor, but he was also a real gentleman. If I whupped him on a drill, he'd simply say: "Way to go."

By my third year with the Steelers, when I became starter, I could hold my own against Joe Greene, Dwight White, or any of our linemen. After practice one day Chuck Noll even told Joe—through the media—that I was "putting welts on him." Of course, he was just trying to motivate Joe.

Normally Chuck saved his dime-store psychology for low-level grunts like myself. I had come to the Steelers as a naïve, highly motivated guy. I wanted to play on a Super Bowl champ. I wanted to win. When Chuck or one of his assistants would ream me out, it would tick me off—plenty. And I'd go back on the field with a really bad attitude and want to hurt people.

Like some other coaches I've had, Chuck determined that this was the best way to motivate me. Looking at my outsized, almost cartoonish body, he probably figured I was just an overgrown puppy—a dumb ol' mutt that could be easily manipulated and motivated.

The irony is that, for much of my career, it worked. I allowed myself to be treated like a dog, or a child, because I wanted to excel—and win—so badly. I also knew that if I wasn't willing to "do what it takes . . . get the job done . . . win at all costs" (or any other typical coach's cliché), there would be someone coming off the sidelines who would. In no time, I'd be out of football and, in Chuck Noll's favorite words, "ready to begin [my] life's work."

It wasn't just me. At one time or another he subjected all of his players to threats and manipulation. Early in his career, Terry Bradshaw was one of Chuck's favorite whipping boys.

"Chuck's personality kept me off balance, which is probably what he wanted," Brad wrote in his book, *Looking Deep*. "One minute I was his prodigal son, the next minute

I was his dog and he was kicking me. Maybe it was his way of keeping control."

I wasn't there during Brad's early years with the Steelers when he struggled, but I heard all the knocks: "Not bright enough to be a quarterback. . . . Great arm, no head. . . . Can't handle the pressure."

Chuck apparently did little to raise the confidence level of his young quarterback, preferring to motivate him via fear and confusion; in several games, the coach shuffled Bradshaw and back-up Terry Hanratty in and out of alternating quarters.

"Chuck and I did not get along," Brad said on the David Letterman show in 1990, seven years after retiring from football. "But you will never have a successful NFL franchise if the coach and the quarterback get along.

"You need somebody who's headstrong and believes in what he's doing out there pulling the trigger, calling the plays, and is so self-assured," Brad continued. "And, if you start trying to interfere, he's going to say: 'Wait a minute. What do you know? Have you ever played in the Super Bowl? Have you ever called a play when its third and 23?!'"

When I came to the Steelers in 1977, Brad had made his share of third-down conversions and had already guided the team to two Super Bowl victories.

I distinctly remember walking onto the field during my first training camp and getting a good look at the man I was being paid to protect.

I had played on a veer attack at South Carolina, with a rollout quarterback, Jeff Grantz, who had a good arm but was known more as a runner; to me, he was a very solid, exceptional quarterback. There I was, huddled with the rookies on the Pittsburgh Steelers, getting instructions from our line coach, when I looked over to where the quarterbacks were tossing lightly to some of the receivers.

I saw Frank Lewis take off on a little stop-and-go: he went 20, 30, 50 yards; Bradshaw sort of pumped once to get some of the kinks out of his arm, and then gently *flicked* a perfect strike to Lewis on the dead run some 80 yards downfield. I had never seen anything like it in my life. One of the veterans walking by said, "Welcome to the NFL, son."

I soon learned to like and respect Brad a great deal, as did most of the other guys, but in the six years that we played together, I never really got to know him that well. He was aloof, likely out of self-protection, and seemed very careful not to reveal too much of himself. I actually felt sorry for him because of all the scrutiny, all the demands on his time, and because, as quarterback, he was always in the eye of the storm. He couldn't go out with his cronies and knock back a few brews without his every move being dissected and analyzed by the Pittsburgh media and the fans.

Brad had complete control of the huddle, but he wasn't dictatorial. He would listen to suggestions from his linemen. He might say: "What do you think about Toss-32 trap, guys? Can you get movement on the noseguard?" And of course we'd grunt back: "Fuck, yeah, we can get movement on the noseguard." Then he'd bark out: "Let's do it!"

Then there were those days that Brad just didn't have it. You could feel it in the huddle on the first series. For some reason, he was mentally distracted and not really into the game. And boy, when Brad played badly, he played *really* badly. Fortunately those off days were rare.

Brad had what Civil War historian Shelby Foote calls "4 A.M. courage." That is, you could wake him at any God-awful hour and he'd be ready to go, no matter what the situation. But Brad could be fearless to a fault. Most of the interceptions he threw were a result of *too* much confidence in his own arm and abilities. Since he could throw at will on most days—in traffic or between two defenders—

he'd often try to overcome the odds. He'd make the wrong—or let's say, the too-bold—tactical play, figuring his sheer talent could get him through. Which it usually did. Later in his career, he took fewer chances, and also learned how to do less on those days when he didn't have it. At that point, he had no peer at his position.

What I particularly admired about Brad was that he never yelled at his offensive line if we missed an assignment and he got sacked, or if he had to rush a ball that was subsequently picked off. He knew we took great pride in our work, and that if we got beat, we felt bad enough and certainly didn't need to get berated by anyone else.

In the late seventies and early eighties, the Steelers were among the league leaders in fewest sacks allowed as well as in most rushing yardage gained. In addition, our pass patterns were predicated on a four-second drop—which meant that our receivers mainly ran 20 to 25 yard routes. Four seconds is a long, long time back there. The NFL average was probably closer to three seconds. That's a huge differential. And we took great pride in that. We all knew that if we wanted to play for the Steelers' offensive line, we had to pass block forever.

There was a definite hierarchy on the Steelers—between superstars such as Brad, Lynn Swann, Jack Lambert, and Joe Greene and the rest of us grunts. We'd party with them on rare occasions if we ran into them, but, for the most part, they kept to themselves. There were obvious reasons: When relatively low-profile guys like myself, Moon Mullins, Gary Dunn, or Tunch Ilkin went out, we might be recognized by fans, who would then buy us drinks, want to talk football, or just brag to their friends that they rubbed shoulders with some real live Steelers. But when those stars went out, it was an event. They could barely eat or drink without being overwhelmed with attention and adulation.

Most of us had our ups and downs with the fans, but

some of the mega-Steelers, Jack Lambert in particular, could be pretty arrogant and even mean to fans, especially when drinking. You never knew if and when Lambert might go off. I don't know if he ever coldcocked someone in a bar, but he certainly could be icy and sarcastic when dealing with the public. In some ways, I could sympathize; people just did not leave him alone. In many ways, Lambert exemplified the Steelers, and the city of Pittsburgh: gritty, gutsy, maybe a little out of control. And as such he was adored by Steeler fans as much, or more, than any other player.

I never disliked Lambert as a person, but I did and still do have certain philosophical differences with him. Before his induction into the Pro Football Hall of Fame in 1989, he wrote an open letter to me in the *Pittsburgh Press* in response to my criticism of the latest wishy-washy NFL directive on steroid use. His letter made some good points, particularly when it came to telling kids the truth about steroids, but then he meandered into self-serving speechify-ing: "Don't tell [young athletes] that in order to be competi-tive, they have to use [steroids]. That would be a lie. As a former 11-year NFL veteran who did not use steroids, I would like to think if anything I was competitive. . . . No drugs. No shortcuts. And no excuses."

I don't want to push the point, but nicotine and alcohol are drugs and maybe as harmful as many illegal ones. For as long as I've known him, Jack has been a chain-smoker and a man who definitely likes his beer. My open letter to Jack would say: "If you want to tell kids the truth, then tell the whole truth and lay off the platitudes and self-righteousness."

Men such as Lambert and Chuck Noll have been deified for so long that when you point out the truth to them, or make them accountable for their actions, they, as well as their fervent supporters, take it personally. No doubt some of these folks will maintain that I was—and am—just jealous. I'd say to them: I may never enter the Hall of Fame, but I do know as well as anyone how the game is played.

Chuck Noll may have treated all of us like dogs, but some of the kennels were a little classier than others. The Steelers, like most NFL teams, did have different sets of rules for different castes of players. But I always felt that most of us on the lower rung rarely let our resentment get out of hand. We acknowledged and even accepted that there was a class system, one standard for grunts and another for officers. A coach would have to be real stupid to ignore that fact; and Chuck Noll may have been cold and manipulative, but he was definitely not stupid.

That's not to say we *never* harbored any resentment, and not only around payday. Many a time—especially during two-a-days (two practices per day)—we'd finish up filthy, bloodied, and aching after the morning session, and then head over to the weight room to put in another hour of heavy lifting. On our way, we might run into Brad, Lynn Swann, Calvin Sweeney, or some of the other guys going out to shoot a fast nine holes of golf between practices. Yeah, we might've wanted to wrap a 2-iron around someone's head at that moment.

There was also some disparity in the media coverage. The Steeler stars seemed to enjoy a free pass with the local press. In Pittsburgh, there's nothing like a superstar on a winning Steeler team. Objectivity was often lost, and these guys were lionized—from a journalistic standpoint—to an inordinate, inappropriate degree. You didn't knock the Steeler superstars during those Super Bowl years, not if you liked your facial features intact. But if a reporter did choose to make a critical comment in a story, usually the grunts were fair game.

My best friends on the Steelers were all men from the

front lines: Gary Dunn from the defensive set, Mike Webster and Tunch Ilkin on offense. Ironically, Tunch had been drafted by the Steelers in the sixth round and then released. When I got hurt in '80, they were short a lineman and had to bring him back. He stuck. I kind of took Tunch under my wing, as Mike Webster had done with me.

That protectiveness seemed to be more prevalent on the offensive line than at other positions. We were all fighting hard for jobs, but there was a sense of community down in the trenches. We performed the dirtiest, most thankless duty, and we took great pride in it. But there was not a great deal of hype or glory attached to it.

We were the shock troops of the infantry, or—to use another military metaphor—the heavy tanks in a ground (and air) assault. We were outfitted in tactical armor that was used as much for weaponry as for our protection. We played with more injuries and suffered more mental abuse than any other soldiers in the field. And we received less approval and far less compensation from our superiors. Self-sacrifice was our credo. (You'd think that the Steeler army, in particular, would be more sympathetic to the men on the front line. After all, our leader, General Noll, had been a messenger guard for the Cleveland Browns in his days as a fighting man.)

While I was closer to the offensive linemen than most other Steelers, the truth is—and this may sound simplistic or bogus—we all got along. Almost without exception, we accepted each other for who we were.

Winning certainly was a factor. It's much easier to be chipper and cheerful when things were going your way. But mainly, I think we were naïve. We believed in the Steelers, in Chuck Noll, and in the Rooneys—especially in the old man, Mr. Art Rooney, Sr.

We called him Mr. Rooney not because he asked us to, certainly not out of sarcasm, but out of respect for the man and the way he treated us. Again, it's sappy to say, but he treated us like family.

After he died, things changed. The Steeler organization became like the rest of the NFL, obsessed with the bottom line (for years it's been one of the lowest-paying teams in the league). Mr. Rooney was one of a handful of original owners who got involved in football because it was fun, not because it looked good on a balance sheet.

There were no racial divisions on the Steelers when I played there, and much of that stemmed from Mr. Rooney. He was as comfortable and expansive with the locker-room attendants as he was with any captain of industry. The only black–white conflicts I recall had to do with what kind of music we should play in the locker room.

Some of the white guys such as Lambert, Dunnie, and myself liked country and Western, while some of the black guys such as Jim Smith and Sidney Thornton only listened to disco-soul sounds. One minute Hank Williams, Jr. or Waylon Jennings would be wafting out of the speakers with their mournful plaints of heartache or heartbreak . . .

"Turn off that shitkicker crap!" Big Sid might scream out, and then he'd twist the dial a couple of notches to the soul station, and Aretha Franklin or Marvin Gaye would be rocking the room . . .

"Get that jungle bunny music outta here!" Gary or I might yell back.

There was also a good deal of sartorial disparity between black and white. In my rookie year we had frequent Dress-Off competitions to determine the team's snazziest dresser. As one who favored Army fatigues and combat boots, I was never in the running.

Yet no man of any color could compete with running back Frenchy Fuqua. The Frenchman would usually win any Dress-Off with some new purple jumpsuit, usually topped off with an oversized cape, plus one of several dozen pair of the most unusual footwear. The kicker, so to speak, was when Frenchy showed up one day with two-inch-high *glass* platform heels filled with goldfish. The goldfish died, and the Dress-Off Award was permanently retired in their honor.

The ethic of those Steeler teams—at least, the guys I was closest to—was work hard and play hard. And we succeeded on all counts. These were the men I depended on to protect my ass; certainly not the old men on the sidelines giving the orders.

When I look back, the only real things for me in my football career were the pain, the combat, and the camaraderie. And, of course, the partying.

The rest of it was crap.

3

ROCK AND ROLL, SEX AND DRUGS

THE SUNDAY NIGHT after a Steeler game—especially a win—was a very heady and hot scene. We'd shower up and usually head straight over to the Pittsburgh Marriott. The place would be crawling with adoring fans, many of whom happened to be beautiful women.

Most of the guys on the offensive line would usually join us, but defensive lineman Gary Dunn was my main co-reveler. He was the only guy who could match me drink for drink, or nearly. Each week, the manager at the Marriott would set up our regular table in the back for us. It would be piled high with platters of shrimp and cheese, as well as huge pitchers of kamikazes (vodka, triple sec, lime concentrate).

One of our favorite practices was to mix kamikazes in our mouths, one ingredient at a time. We'd lean our heads back over the bar, and the bartender would pour in ice, vodka, and the rest. Then, with our mouths filled to overflowing, we'd try to quickly stand up while swallowing the entire concoction. I say "try" because it'd be a real effort to stand up without falling down on those rubbery legs. After two or three of these, it felt a lot like getting blindsided by a 290-pound defensive lineman at full tilt.

We'd often rope in a few willing, and occasionally unwilling ("Here, drink this . . .") civilians from the surrounding throng to join in our fun. What did we care? All the food and liquor were on the house. The house was smart, too, figuring it was good business to have real live Steelers in such close proximity to the regular paying customers. And, of course, any of the women who wanted to rub shoulders, or other body parts, with a couple of young studs knew where they could find us.

Which they usually did.

It was like the howling of the gladiators after their victory. We'd be releasing steam after surviving the battle, just glad to be young, vital, alive. And at the end of the evening's revelry there'd be six or seven girls clustered around our table to choose from, if we were so inclined.

I was under no illusions. I never thought that these women were interested in me because I was such a scintillating raconteur or for my thorough knowledge of military history.

Still and all, it led to a very skewed perspective for a young man to have women throw themselves at us. Even then, I knew how shallow it was. And sort of disturbing. No matter how rude or crass we became—not to anyone in particular, but just rowdy boys in general—these women would still want to go home with us. Because we were celebrities. Because we were Steelers.

Being Steelers also kept us out of jail.

On at least two instances, both occurring on the road after a night of carousing, we escaped the wrath of the law—and probably some time in the pokey—because of who we were. For the same offense, any of the so-called civilians who'd partied with us earlier would have likely been locked up.

The first time, in 1980, I was behind the wheel. I had just spent four weeks on injured reserve with a dislocated foot in a cast while watching the team struggle to a .500 record. I was frustrated as hell that I couldn't play. I couldn't even work out. Probably the most productive thing I did during that time was install a new brush guard on my Chevy Blazer.

One Saturday night I was out partying particularly hard, pub crawling (or driving) all over town in my Blazer, downing shots and beers wherever I went. Finally, heading home in the wee hours, it struck me that there were too many STOP signs in Pittsburgh. It really pissed me off that I had to constantly brake for all these damn signs.

It was probably the culmination of frustration and anger I felt as a result of not playing and not contributing. Though I wasn't on cycle at the time, it felt like a 'roid attack—moments of sheer aggression precipitated by a large dosage or a lengthy cycle of steroid use. I'd had several of those in the past.

Whatever it was, I had soon psyched myself into a blind rage. Using my new brush guard as a battering ram, I proceeded to knock down every single irritating STOP sign that I found on my way home.

It didn't take a law-enforcement genius to follow the trail of broken signs to my door, especially with my truck parked well up on the sidewalk in front of my town-house.

Fortunately the young officer who came to investigate the following morning was somewhat sympathetic to my hungover condition. I ended up paying for the signs; and, other than having to deal with my acute embarrassment, the case was considered closed.

The strike year of 1982 was another very frustrating time for all of us. The players' slogan was "55 percent!" (of the gross), which we of course did not even approach in the eventual settlement. But we did squeeze out some minimal benefits, including increased severance pay. It was an eye-opening experience for me, observing firsthand how the owners manipulated the issues—and the media—for their own purposes.

One night, after a NFLPA (National Football League Players Association) meeting chaired by executive member Tom Condon, guard for the Kansas City Chiefs, we left the Greentree Marriott for a bar in Shadyside to blow off a little steam. Afterwards Gary Dunn took Tom and me back to my place in his jeep.

On the way, Gary's own anger and disillusionment came to a flash point: He drove us in and around the side streets of Pittsburgh at high speeds, including several blocks on the sidewalks. Tom and I were mighty glad to see the lights of my townhouse complex in suburban Bridgeville.

As we ascended the long hill leading up to the complex, Gary suddenly jerked the jeep to the right and clipped every mailbox on the street. He didn't miss a one. By the time we got to my apartment, we were laughing and whooping like banshees. Several minutes later, a policeman was at my door.

"Who's vehicle is parked outside?" the officer asked. Gary sheepishly raised his hand.

"Have you been drinking, Mr. Dunn?" the officer asked, immediately recognizing Gary.

While tilting back and forth, Gary's reply was honest, if not entirely circumspect: "Do I look like a sober man to you?"

The officer continued with his line of questioning.

"Mr. Dunn, did you run over all the mailboxes on this street?"

Gary looked the policeman in the eye—or tried to—while he weaved. He said: "If I had a tank, I would have run over the houses, too."

Gary got off with a simple warning. They accepted his offer to buy each homeowner a new mailbox, and everyone walked away happy. Thankfully, in both of these instances—as well as on many more occasions when we should not have been driving at all—no one was hurt.

But hey, officer, I'm a Steeler.

Years later, when I went to Alcoholics Anonymous and heard so many tragic stories of drunk drivers, I realized that a lot of other folks were not as fortunate.

The strike year also introduced me to the art of the tailgate party. Tailgating is when fans get together before and sometimes after a game in the stadium parking lot and pig out on prepared or barbecued food, drink beer, and drink a lot more beer. Since I was usually playing, I had missed out on the joys of tailgating. As an initiation, Dunnie and I drove to Penn State for the homecoming game against Syracuse. After a few hours of tailgating our big old tails off, we headed into Beaver Stadium (you can imagine the humor we found in that), and later tailgated a little more.

By the next day, on the drive home, we were both nursing two humungous hangovers. We turned on the radio (low) for some soothing music, and heard: "Bradshaw is back to pass, and he finds Stallworth for the first down."

What?!?

Gary and I looked at each other in a sweaty panic: Could we have missed the end of the strike? Could the season have resumed without us knowing about it? Were our careers over?

We soon realized that it was a repeat broadcast of an old Super Bowl. Oh, thank you, Lord.

Most off-seasons I spent some time in Florida visiting Gary, and I can remember at least one other memorable drive of ours. An inquisitive Coral Gables police officer pulled Dunnie's van over, citing "mysterious rocking" in the back. Dunnie explained that the rocking was simply caused by me practicing a bodybuilding pose called the "crab."

"Would you like to see it?" Gary asked the trooper.

The cop said, "Sure."

And, sure enough, I jumped out of the van, screaming, "Do you want to see it!?! Well, here it is!" I then showed him three or four of my most peeled poses, veins and muscles bulging out to here.

"Do you want to see any more?!" I yelled. The officer just told us to get back in the car and get the hell out of there.

During the regular season, I went through what I called my "descending ritual" on the Monday after a game (assuming I woke up in my own three-level Bridgeville townhouse): The alarm would wake me up around 10 A.M. in the third-floor bedroom; I'd walk down to the middle floor and grab a six-pack out of the fridge; then I'd descend to the lower floor (the basement Jacuzzi having been preset to heat up at 9 A.M.), where I'd gently lower my creaking bones into the tub. With a beer in one hand and a remote control in the other, I'd soak away my soreness for virtually the entire day.

Often, when I think back to those wild, carefree days, I can't believe that guy was me. At the time, however, it did seem like a great life. What could be better? Getting paid to perform in a sport that I would have played for nothing. Blowing off some steam with my good buddies after "work." And meeting any number of beautiful, agreeable women.

During the heart of my NFL career, I was not interested in getting married or even forging any long-term relationships. Football was my life, my wife, and my mistress. I was out there to gladiate (if that's a verb), and I was very, very serious about it. That's why I took steroids, to be the best I could be. And, in many cases, I looked at the available women as spoils of war.

I was also instinctively wary of romantic entanglements. I had seen too many guys getting involved with women who were more interested in the money than their honey, so to speak.

As it turned out, I should have been even warier.

During the 1983 season, I was once again drowning my sorrows in a local pub because of a knee injury. An attractive, if overly aggressive, woman suggested I take her home. Which I did. But since I was so drunk, I don't recall what, if anything, happened.

A few weeks later, I returned to the same watering establishment. As I was becoming such a good customer, some of the staff informed me that the female companion I had recently met there had been "familiar" with most of the bar's clientele.

Basically, she came onto anything with slacks and a jockstrap.

During that off-season, I was in the midst of negotiating my most lucrative—and, unknowingly, final—NFL contract with the Steelers. A few weeks before training camp, the woman from the bar told me that she was pregnant and I was definitely the father. While I had major doubts of that fact, I felt sorry for her and gave her some money.

A year later, I received notification of a paternity suit filed in Pittsburgh family court. I had to submit to a blood test and, in the course of the proceedings, confront the woman and the child.

The mother gave me the little girl to hold. She did not look like me, but who could tell at that age? For a moment, I contemplated the idea of having a child, a daughter. It wasn't entirely unpleasant. But I decided to wait for the results before I thought too much of Sunday outings, braces, and college tuition.

The blood test came back negative. I was relieved. From that moment on, I became much more cautious and "protective" in dealing with women.

There have been conflicting tales on steroids and sex. All steroids used by athletes are derivatives of the male sex hormone testosterone, which means one's libido is usually affected. A few male users have experienced a diminished sex drive. For me, and most of the guys I knew, steroids were an aphrodisiac.

A friend of mine, a weightlifter, told me about the time he competed in a local meet during a testosterone cypionate cycle.

"I had just put my supersuit on," he said, "and this beautiful, buxom woman in a tight dress walks by. All of a sudden I feel this excruciating pain in my groin. I had apparently popped a hard-on, and because these suits are so tight, my erection was pushing against the fabric—which is like rubber and doesn't give at all. I had to take off the suit and wait until my hard-on subsided."

Steroids definitely increased my interest in sex. When I was on cycle, my entire body became electric. Every nerve ending and organ seemed *pumped*.

Reduced to simpler terms: I became one horny young man.

Like most people, I'd always enjoyed sex. But I'd never been consumed by a need for it. I was not the type of guy who went out on a Friday night simply to get laid. I could have just as good a time hanging out with my buddies, downing shots, swapping stories.

Other than on the football field, I have tried to remain in complete control of my life. As such, I tried not to let my little head do the thinking for the big head. However, I soon found that when I cycled steroids, it became a lot more imperative to be with a woman. I was no longer in complete control of all my bodily organs.

I was never purposely crass about it. I never grabbed or pawed strange women in public places. But I do remember honing in like a laser beam whenever a really good-looking lady passed by.

Toward the end of a typical cycle, one of the drugs I'd take to restimulate the natural testosterone processes was human chorionic gonadatropin (HCG). HCG is a fertility hormone made from pregnant women's urine. No kidding. The drug is know to further enhance one's sex drive—and even performance. For one thing, it will give a man some serious stamina. Most guys who use it are weightlifters, but I know others who take HCG just so they can impress their girlfriends.

HCG, a crystalized solution that's mixed with water and injected directly into the gluteus maximus, is obviously not for the fainthearted. And while no major side effects have been discovered thus far, the research has been minimal. I would hate to think that young people would possibly endanger their health in any way for a few kinky kicks.

Some doctors have even linked HCG to dilated cardiomyopathy. While I haven't seen any direct evidence, I have read of a connection between heart disease and some of the Soviet athletes who took HCG as part of their weight-training regimen. Again, because of the absence of real research, we just don't know the precise effects.

I can probably say with some surety that offensive

linemen were—and are—more likely to use steroids to enhance (football) performance than players at other positions. The reasons are simple: Your job relies more on physical strength than any other. Your basic purpose is to push someone in a direction that he doesn't want to go. And when these reluctant someones are 270, 280, even 300 pounds of speed and muscle, you've got a real occupational hazard.

Technique may keep you around for awhile. Knowledge of tactics is essential. Certainly quickness is an asset. But you cannot last in the National Football League as an effective run or pass blocker without brute, out-of-this-world strength. And there are two main ways to build strength: weightlifting and steroids. If you combine the two, the results will be extraordinary.

Without naming names, I can state unequivocally that during my time in Pittsburgh 75 percent of the Steeler offensive line took anabolic-androgenic steroids at one time or another. Disgruntled players throughout the league called us the "Steroid Team," as if performance-enhancing drugs were the sole reason for our success.

The fact is, our AAS usage was the same—give or take—as most of the NFL teams at that time.

Pat Donovan, a Dallas Cowboy offensive lineman who retired in 1983 after nine years in the NFL, has said: "In my last five or six years [steroid use] ran as high as 60 to 70 percent on the Cowboys' offensive and defensive lines." And in 1985, while playing for the Raiders, defensive end Lyle Alzado said, "On some teams, between 75 and 90 percent of all [players] use steroids."

What the Steelers had was one of the most advanced strength programs under Lou Rickey, and some of the most dedicated, hard-working athletes in or out of football. When the NFL began its Strongest Man Competition in 1980, the

Steelers dominated it: Mike Webster won it in 1980, with Jon Kolb and Steve Furness second and sixth; in 1981, Kolbie won, and I came in third; and in 1982, Rick Donnalley won, with me in second and Craig Wolfley in fourth.

While I would estimate that about 50 percent of the team in the power positions experimented with anabolic-androgenic steroids, an even greater number took amphetamines on Sunday before a game. The use of amphetamines was much more open during the early years of pro football; there are confirmed stories of cups or cookie jars in several locker rooms, sitting out for all to see, from which interested players could scoop up however many pills they wanted.

Since the offensive line on the Steelers were so close, we discussed anything and everything. Among ourselves— away from the coaches and the media—we talked about our feminine conquests, our jobs, and about our drug use.

It was like group therapy. Most of us were just learning about anabolic-androgenic steroids. They seemed like wonderful new toys, and if one of us discovered a more effective drug, we were eager to share it with the others.

Some of my Steeler teammates and other serious weight-lifting friends would occasionally gather around my kitchen table and discuss our mood swings or our latest 'roid attacks. Most of us agreed that the juice made us more sexually aware men, though the levels of arousal varied among us.

There was considerably less variance, however, when it came to aggression. In all cases, when we took steroids our aggressiveness got turned way up. Which, of course, is another reason why coaches choose to look the other way. They're constantly yelling at the players to "hit harder!" Or: "Be more aggressive!" And here is that magical pill (or injection) that could do just that.

Anabolic-androgenic steroids and amphetamines definitely increased our levels of aggression. Some of us, myself included, would use marijuana to take the edge off of the 'roid rage and/or the speed rush we might experience; it also tended to smooth out the gladiator mentality, which might not be appropriate in a social setting. Other than the occasional joint, however, I was not really an ardent recreational drug user.

Like many of my generation, I did experiment with most drugs—usually once, out of curiosity—including mushrooms, acid, quaaludes, opium, ecstasy, and cocaine. Some I enjoyed more than others, but I never did any of them regularly. I was too focused on football and didn't want any additional distractions.

The one drug that left me especially cold was cocaine. It didn't do much other than make my heart race and my nose burn. Many of my teammates—some at Pittsburgh, more at Tampa Bay—were into coke fairly heavily. The combination of cocaine and steroids would have most of these guys bouncing off of walls, barstools, bar patrons—you name it. Needless to say, it was not the most peaceable union.

As for amphetamines, which can make you hyper and aggressive all by their lonesome, I used them maybe three times in my entire pro career. The first time was in 1978, my second year with the Steelers, when my basic function was that of a messenger guard—ferrying the plays in from Chuck Noll to Terry Bradshaw.

It was a Monday night game against the Oilers, and I wanted a little extra fuel for the national TV audience—in this case, two black beauties. Sometime in the second quarter, Chuck yelled the play in my ear, "I-84 Trap Pass," and I eagerly trotted out onto the field to inform my teammates. Which I did, of course. All except one.

It seemed that I had told the play to everyone except our

quarterback, Bradshaw, who instead calls out, "Flow-37." We're about to break huddle when it dawned on me—even in my "beaned out" state—that something was amiss. I leaned over and whispered to Brad, "That's not the play." He laughed and called a time out. You can be sure, however, that Chuck Noll was not laughing.

As you may guess from that episode, amphetamines—speed, beauties, beenies, beanies, greenies—made me goofy. I couldn't think straight. If they had worked for me, like they did for many players throughout the league, I probably would've taken them more frequently.

As I mentioned, a speed or 'roid rush was perceived by most of us as a positive thing, a belief tacitly shared by our coaches. The way I figured, I was getting paid to explode on the line of scrimmage, and if I occasionally exploded in my car out of rage—often, when caught in rush-hour traffic, I'd feel like ripping the steering wheel off its column—I shouldn't take the ups and downs too seriously.

Fortunately, I was able to keep my aggressions confined within the dimensions of a football field—for the most part. But there were moments when I acknowledged that there might be a real down side to this combativeness in civilian life.

At 21, after having completed only two steroid cycles, I got into a brutal bar fight in Florida and nearly killed a man. It was after my first season on injured reserve. Needing to blow off some steam, some of my college buddies and I piled into the Cutlass Salon that I had bought with my bonus money, turned on the fuzzbuster, and drove down to Jacksonville to watch Pitt play Clemson in the Gator Bowl. The night before the game, my friends—who were all football players—and I went out with some guys from the Pitt team. The smallest guy in our group weighed 215 pounds.

We had been in this bar for only a few minutes—it was the second stop on our Jacksonville pub crawl and we had maybe a couple of Heinekens—when my roommate, Jerome, comes over to me and says, "Steve, there are these guys over there who need a real beating."

I was stunned. Jerome, who had been the teenage national powerlifting champ, was the sweetest guy you'd ever want to meet, big as a polar bear with the temperament of a teddy bear. I had lived with the guy for two years and had never even heard him raise his voice.

"C'mon, Jerome," I said, "There're lots of ladies around. Don't worry about these idiots. Relax."

No more than 30 seconds later, two of these Southern gentlemen were in both of our faces giving us a load of redneck rudeness about our lineage and something about our pussy Yankee butts. I had a little buzz from the beers going, and was now in no mood to listen to any more of this cracker crap. I had heard enough of it at South Carolina from my coaches.

"Okay, guys," I said, "you want us, you got us." And we took a walk outside.

Meanwhile, I'm thinking, these two regular-sized guys must really be wacko. I mean, they see the bulk on us; I was about 270 then, and Jerome was around 265. What could they possibly be thinking—or drinking?

And then I saw that we'd been set up.

Out in the parking lot, these two weasels were flanked in a semi-circle by 10 of their buddies. Some of them were holding broken beer bottles. Jerome and I looked at each other—kind of like Butch and Sundance—and went, "Oh, shit." But we weren't about to back down. Besides, these guys didn't know that we had three other extra-large fellows who were on their way out.

I finally said, "Well, ladies, if you'd like to take your bra and panties off, we can get down to it." One of them came over and pushed me, and I just lost it. I threw him to the ground and began whaling on him. At least five of his friends jumped on my back and start playing a drum solo on my head with their fists and feet. It was chaos out there, really nuts. The crack of fists on bone, guys flying through the air.

Soon bodies were being picked off of me like flies. Jerome and my three other buddies had arrived like the cavalry and were soon tossing these guys all over the lot—really kicking the crap out of their shitkicking asses. It might've been five against 12, but our five were about as serious as they get. As football players, most of us were used to getting hit. Some of us even liked it.

Prior to that night, I don't think I had ever hit a guy in the face. But facing off against one of the original instigators from the bar, I was so consumed by anger that I swung at the guy's head with all my might.

I missed.

Then I really got mad. The next three times I connected—full on—and he went down like a rag doll. He lay there slumped on the ground, with his eyes rolled back in his head. I assumed he was dead.

The thought that you may have just killed a man will sober you up real fast. It was the worst feeling I'd ever had. I was just filled with waves of nausea and regret. Then I heard police sirens blaring in the distance.

I'm thinking, Oh, God, oh, God.

As it turned out, the guy had simply gotten all his lights turned off for several minutes. But those few minutes were easily the scariest in my life, much more so than being told that I had a life-threatening illness.

I decided at that point that I never wanted to hit anyone—other than on a football field—again. I was a danger to myself and definitely to others. The monster that I had created through weight training and steroids was not meant for hand-to-hand combat with civilians.

Subsequently, I've walked away from more fights in my life than I can count. You'd be amazed at the things people would say to me—figuring I was either too big or too dumb to do anything about it. I guess it's human nature to want to challenge the big guy, though some of it may have been just plain jealousy. There I was, with a pretty impressive physique, not the ugliest dude in the world, making pretty good dough, playing on a world-champion football team in a town where football was right up there with family, flag, and country (and beer). I was a big target.

Problems often arose when the young women in the vicinity might've been paying more attention to us than to some of the other fellows around. And sometimes, particularly with their beer muscles on, I was challenged by guys simply looking to drop me a few pegs.

It's a wonder, particularly on cycle, that my teammates and I didn't get into more fistfights.

On or off cycle, some of my Steeler teammates and I spent a good deal of time discussing various "stacks," or drug combinations. We sounded like a bunch of pharmacists talking shop.

"Two cc's of liquid Dianabol," I might suggest. "Injected right into the glute [gluteus maximus, or buttock]."

"What do you know about Winstrol V [an injectable water-based steroid that Ben Johnson tested positive for]?" someone might ask.

"Deca-Durabolin has a nice kick," another might recommend.

"How 'bout testosterone cypionate?"

By the end of my football career, in 1985, I was taking four different shots twice a week, each containing one of the above steroids.

We also talked about some of the noticeable side effects.

Almost all of us experienced, in addition to more productive training and increased libido, some problems with acne, oily skin, water retention, and, of course, irritability.

Sometimes we might even adjourn from the kitchen table to the bedroom, where we'd inject some of these drugs into our buttocks or thighs. On occasion some nurses we were friendly with would come by and shoot us up.

However, we had few "shooting parties" that compared with those described by Tommy Chaikin—a player from my alma mater, South Carolina—in Rick Telander's exposé of college football, *The Hundred Yard Lie*:

> Seven or eight of us heavy users would get together in a dorm room and start shooting each other up. Guys would show up with their bottles, and there'd be a lot of chatter: I shoot you, you shoot me. We all enjoyed it. I had boxes of syringes that I got from certain pharmacies in Columbia for twenty bucks a hundred. We never used the same needles twice, I can tell you that. We tried to be careful how we injected each other, too, but sometimes you'd hit the sciatic nerve or something, and the guy's legs would buckle. I mean, none of us were doctors or anything. But we were needle happy. We would have injected ourselves with anything if we thought it would make us big.

Chaikin, who is a few years younger than me, has experienced virtually every side effect in the book as a result of his steroid use.

My buddies and I were willing to try anything that would make us bigger, stronger, faster. As for future consequences or side effects, they were irrelevant. We were young and invincible. In those days, we felt nothing could hurt us.

The first documented account of steroid use in professional football appeared in *Sports Illustrated* in the fabled summer of 1969, around the time of Woodstock, men landing on the moon, the Mets heading for their first pennant.

Dave Kocourek, an offensive end with the San Diego Chargers in the early sixties, claimed that "this anabolic steroid business [in the NFL] must have started on the Chargers around 1963," coinciding with the team's hiring of Alvin Roy, a Baton Rouge gym owner, as the league's first "strength coach."

In the article, Kocourek claimed that Roy and the Chargers were passing out Dianabol to virtually all of the players:

> One day, I asked Alvin and Sid Gillman, our coach, if the team physician had okayed these pills. They gave me sort of a vague answer. I don't remember what the answer was, but I do remember that it didn't satisfy me. As it happened, I lived next door to a physician and I asked him about anabolic steroids.
>
> The doctor told me, "Listen, Dave, I don't think these things were intended for people who do the kind of work you people do. I think they were made for Milquetoast-type guys, people who sit in chairs all day long and never get a chance to build any healthy muscular tissue."
>
> I told the other guys this and a lot of them quit taking them. Don't get me wrong. It wasn't ever any great big deal, or any cause for rebellion or mutiny. But a lot of the fellows just started throwing them away.

It's also interesting to note how limited the physician's knowledge of the drugs was then; today, after nearly thirty years of common usuage in the NFL, doctors still don't know a hell of a lot more on the subject. Their continued ignorance goes to show how disposable athletes really are.

Hall of Fame offensive guard Ron Mix, who played with the Chargers in 1963, confirmed Kocourek's account:

Alvin [Roy] had been an assistant coach of one of our Olympic weightlifting teams and he learned a secret from "them Rooskies," he informed us while explaining the virtue of Dianabol.

He did not say that the pills were steroids, only that taking them would help us assimilate protein, "the building blocks of muscle." We had taken the pills three times a day for five weeks when [Kocourek's] family doctor advised him he shouldn't take it for extended periods of time. When the rest of us heard that, most stopped. But for many, the prospect of being stronger was too intoxicating, the hope for an advantage too enticing, the fear of failure too great; and they continued. The club continued to offer Dianabol to the team as long as I was in San Diego. Civilian casualties were acceptable.

Chuck Noll testified before a Senate subcommittee that he knew virtually nothing about his players' steroid use in three decades of coaching. In fact, he stated for the record that only three of his players ever tested positive for steroids—"none of which [sic] made the team"—as if this was the extent of the problem as far as he knew it.

However, Chuck Noll was an assistant coach for the San Diego Chargers in 1963 (as were Al Davis and John Madden)—the exact time frame cited by both Dave Kocourek and Ron Mix in which Dianabol was freely dispensed. Did he turn a blind eye to the situation? I'd think only a fool could be unaware of such widespread steroid use. And Chuck, as I've mentioned, was nobody's fool.

In 1983, during Steeler training camp, I pulled a hamstring running a 40-yard dash. Chuck reamed me out in front of the entire squad, blaming my injury squarely on performance-enhancing drugs. "All you want to do is bodybuild and take steroids!" he screamed at me.

This was a full two years before I admitted my steroid

usage in *Sports Illustrated*, which was one of the first times that an *active* football player had ever confessed in print to taking steroids in order to become a bigger, stronger, more effective athlete.

So, prior to my public admission, Chuck Noll was convinced—rightly, I might add—that I was using steroids. Evidently he was not as blind or ignorant to the steroid issue as he would have the politicians and the public believe.

Instead of accepting any responsibility for perpetuating a corrupt system, Chuck chose to blame the players, testifying that steroid use in the NFL "has grown from small doses to mega-doses in pursuit of mega-bucks." Chuck, in essence, accused the players of greed, while ignoring the billions of dollars made off of their efforts by the league poobahs and owners.

In truth, Chuck never encouraged steroid use on the Steelers, but he conveniently and most definitely turned his head to it. What disappoints me most about Chuck Noll is that he absolves himself of any knowledge or approval—no matter how tacit. Nor does he acknowledge the pressure that players are under to play the game. It's as if we're all interchangeable foot soldiers. One goes down; another one takes his place.

Is it fair or realistic to simply blame the troops? How can one reasonably expect soldiers, on their own initiative, to put down their weapons unconditionally? If the generals want to wage a win-at-all-costs war, how can the grunts change the face of battle? And if one side has all the guns, and the other side has bows and arrows . . . well, it may be admirable to fight so purely, but it's also suicidal.

Obviously Chuck Noll is not alone in this attitude. Virtually every coach lives and works under the same belief system. And virtually every coach turns his head to the drug problem: if not steroids, then certainly painkillers and amphetamines.

It isn't only the NFL. I began using steroids in college. How many kids today are using these drugs in high school, or even earlier? A study by the U.S. Department of Health and Human Service estimates that 250,000 adolescents in this country are using anabolic steroids. Other studies claim twice that number.

What should we do—blame the kids?

4

TALKING
TRASH AND
TACTICS

THOUGH WE CONVERSED freely among ourselves, few Steelers went in for mouthing off, talking trash, or "dissing" (disrespecting) an opponent. We were world champions. It seemed bush and unprofessional to jabber obscenities or anything else at our counterparts across the scrimmage line.

Personally, I never thought it was sound strategy to try and win a talking war. I preferred to let my helmet and shoulder pads speak for me. However, there were several guys I played against—such as Mike St. Clair of Cleveland and Cincinnati, Bubba Baker of the Lions and Cardinals, Houston's Robert Brazile—who were known for trying to verbally intimidate an opponent during the course of a game. Nothing too clever or imaginative, just the usual string of scatological bombast, such as: "Your sorry ass is mine." And: "I'm gonna git you, sucka." Or: "Don't come around here with that weak shit, you pussy mother."

For some reason, Brazile really had it in for Chuck Noll

and would take every opportunity to taunt him directly. If, for example, the Oiler defense stopped us on a key third-down situation, he'd look over to the Steeler sidelines and yell, "How'd you like that one, Chuck?!" (As if *Brazile* was responsible for stopping *Noll*.) I don't think Chuck ever heard him, but we always got a kick out of our coach getting razzed.

Dan Hampton of the Bears was more of a whiner than a talker, with most of his plaints directed toward the officials. He was constantly complaining to the refs, begging for holding penalties. Other players referred to him as a cry-baby, but I thought it was simply smart football. I played pretty well against Dan through most of my career, and we seemed to respect each other's abilities. The only time we got into a little "something," it was my fault.

At the end of my career I played with the Tampa Bay Buccaneers and in 1985, Chicago came into Tampa on their way to the Super Bowl. It was the middle of the game on a scorching-hot day; Dan and I found ourselves in the middle of a pile. While on the ground, in the heat of the moment, I yanked him by the back of his helmet. He got up stomping mad and yelled at me: "You're a better football player than that!" I sheepishly replied: "I know, but we're 0-4." Dan was probably so surprised by my response that he forgot to complain to the official (who didn't see the infraction).

The few discussions I initiated with an opponent were usually to compliment him; I might say, "Good play" or "Solid hit, man." But if someone cheap-shotted me—with a late hit or a chop block—then I'd be in his face plenty. (In those days, our biggest fear was that one chop block—where the guy goes right for your knees, easily the most vulnerable body part of a football player—could end a career. One hit to the knee, one snap of some bone or cartilage, and you're out of football for good. The chop block was subsequently outlawed by the league.)

I might even threaten him with some choice language of my own: "Try that again, and I'll end your fucking career, you scumbag!"

Robert Jackson, a Cleveland linebacker, was a real cheap-shot artist known for taking a lot of late hits. Others with notorious reputations were Doug Dieken of the Browns and Ron Heller, an offensive lineman for the Eagles (and a former Bucs teammate).

Cheap shots were one thing. Intimidation was, of course, acceptable. On the Steelers, we certainly used our share of strongarm tactics early in a game—maybe ring a few extra bells—in order to establish team superiority. Of course, four Super Bowl rings carried with them a certain built-in resonance.

We were accused of one subtle "strongarm" tactic, however, that was not what it appeared. The Pittsburgh offensive line was one of the first teams of the modern era to tailor their jerseys with short, tight sleeves. Because most of us had arms like barrels, we were charged with trying to intimidate our opponents—both with our bulging biceps and with our obliviousness to discomfort (wearing short sleeves without a sweatshirt in subzero temperatures). The fact is, those short, tight sleeves—in which we used double-backed masking tape to keep the jersey snug against the shoulder pads—were more of an artful strategic device. They prevented defensive linemen from using our uniforms as handles; if they couldn't easily grab onto us, they couldn't easily move us.

We were certainly not above using other forms of gamesmanship, including the insidious "influence play."

The Steelers always finished up the exhibition season with a game against the Cowboys. In 1983 we played them down in Irving, Texas, on a typically bearishly hot day. Most of the regulars just wanted to get through the game with a minimum of effort and a complete absence of injury.

But some of the marginal guys out there were fighting for a job or looking to make a name at our expense. I was matched up that day against one of those hungry guys, Bob Smerek, a backup defensive tackle. Bob was getting a little too energetic, and I decided I needed a way to cool his ardor: the influence play.

Defensive linemen are taught to read the offensive lineman's head—it's like a "tell" in poker that gives away a player's hand—so that if I move my head to the outside, chances are I'm going outside to "hook" them, and they can anticipate accordingly. Some offensive linemen will occasionally try to "deke" an opponent by moving the head in the opposite direction to which he's going. It's such a subtle movement that the defensive player often isn't aware (even after the fact) that he's been influenced.

So, to mellow out Mr. Smerek, I threw a barely perceptible head move to the outside, and sure enough, he swallowed the bait. He broke to the outside, while our running back ran through a hole the size of Texas for an easy ten-yard gain. You could see the frustration in the poor guy's eyes, and he didn't even have a clue to how he had been beaten. I felt so bad for the guy that I told him: "the influence play." He smiled, almost relieved that it wasn't any physical mistake on his part.

Then I did it to him again, and we gained 12 yards.

The influence play, surprisingly, was not used as much as you'd think. Physically rough, mentally tough football players didn't like to use such subtle tricks; they preferred to steamroll their opponents with sheer strength rather than try and trick them with finesse (although, invariably, it was the guys who relied on some guile who lasted longest in the league).

The Steeler line *loved* playing in particularly adverse—usually freezing or snowy—conditions. The worse the better. Many of us were brought up in the North, and we were accustomed to cold winters. From a tactical stand-point, we also felt that it gave us a distinct advantage (and not just with the short-sleeved jerseys). In bad weather, the offensive lineman has the edge because he knows the cadence and the direction of the play; the defender has to react, and if the footing or vision is poor, that reaction will be slowed.

On a bus ride over to Cleveland, before a big game against the Browns, Mike Webster and I tried to remember the words to Patton's famous "weather prayer." Rather than try and influence the gods for fair weather (as General Patton requested of the skies over the Ardennes in 1944 during the winter offensive), we were angling for an all-out blizzard. With Cleveland's Municipal Stadium looming in the near distance, we attempted to lead the team in a mock version of Patton's prayer, which *actually* goes like this:

> *Almighty and most merciful father, we humbly beseech thee of great goodness to restrain the immoderate weather with which we've had to contend. Grant us fair weather for battle. Graciously harken to us that as soldiers who call upon thee that armed with thy power we may advance from victory to victory and crush the oppression and wickedness of our enemies and establish thy justice among men and nations. Amen!*

As a result of that misguided chaplain with the chicken feathers from South Carolina, I've never held much truck with mixing religion and football. But, with the infamous Dawg Pound barking and howling for our hides, we'd accept any form of positive intervention, divine or otherwise.

As it turned out, it had already rained prior to game time, and the field was somewhat soggy. I mention that because it became a key factor in my humiliation before 80,000 screaming fans, as well as my teammates.

Nearing the goal line, the Steelers often used a formation in which Ray Pinney, an offensive tackle, would line up at tight end. We had agreed in the meeting room earlier that if Ray ever scored a touchdown, he'd give me the ball and I'd dunk it over the goalpost. (As one of the better basketball players on the team, I was known for my leaping—and dunking—ability.) Sure enough, Ray made the catch in the end zone and happily tossed the ball to me. I palmed it in one hand and ran up to the goalpost for my leaping, shining moment. But on the way up, I slipped on the wet grass (or at least that's the excuse I later gave) and barely *pinned* the ball on the crossbar. The "Pound," which had been quiet after the touchdown, began jeering and barking anew. (I caught even more abuse on Tuesday from my linemates when we viewed the game film.)

We did win the game, which may or may not say something about the power of prayer, but it was not exactly my proudest moment.

On the offensive line, we always felt that real football—down, dirty, in-your-face kind of football—was fourth and one, or fourth and goal. That's where all the controlled violence and drama are concentrated into a few moments of hand-to-hand, pad-to-pad combat. In trench warfare, there isn't much room for illusion, and not much margin for error. You either get it done or you don't.

However, there was one goal-line situation I can recall, against the Rams, in which we tried to fool our opponents with a little magic trick: Chuck Noll asked us to hide a 300-pound man. The Steelers had a play called "extra guard right" in which we added another lineman for some more blocking. The extra guard was usually 5' 11", 300-pound Tyrone McGriff (whom we cruelly nicknamed Tie-load McDump for his rotund physique). We had run this play several times that day with some success, and were planning to run it again toward the end of the game when the

Rams called a time out. In order to conceal the play from the Rams, we tried to conceal Tyrone from them. So, throughout the time out, Tyrone squatted in the huddle directly behind Webbie and myself. We couldn't stop giggling as we tried to jostle for the best angle of obstruction.

Another proud moment in Steeler history.

One of the things in my pro career that I am proudest of is that I never received an unsportsmanlike conduct penalty. I played hard, very hard, but always—in my mind—fairly and honorably. And I felt the same could be said about the Steelers.

Rival players or coaches, of course, might disagree with that assessment.

"Chuck Noll was the most brutal coach in history," said Jerry Glanville, former head coach of the Houston Oilers—a division rival of the Steelers—and most recently of the Atlanta Falcons. "When he was on top, he had his players whip you like a hound. In the early Eighties [the Steelers] ground Warren Moon's head into the dirt, you needed a drill to get it out."

Of course, Jerry might not be the most objective guy, particularly when it comes to Chuck Noll.

"I had a face injury once," Glanville has joked. "The doctors wanted to cut. The trouble was I'd never smile again. Just like Chuck Noll."

Jerry Glanville and Chuck Noll have a bit of a history, little of it cordial. Perhaps their most famous interaction—which Mark Kram described for *Esquire*—was a postgame "chat" at midfield in 1987:

> *The ritualistic shaking of hands (the Steelers had been all but put in body bags) takes place; but Noll won't let the hand go. "You tried to hurt us. Your guys coming over, jumping on people like that, you're going to get your ass in*

trouble." Jerry tried to free himself, and there's Noll croak-
ing, "I'm serious!"

That's Chuck—serious, all right. But I can't recall a time
that he ever told us to go out and hurt anyone.

We did, of course, have a few guys on our team—such as
Jack Lambert, L.C. Greenwood, Mel Blount, and Donnie
Shell—who were known for playing particularly "physical
football."

What does that mean exactly?

I've heard that phrase a lot over the past several years.
During our heyday, the Steelers were frequently referred to
by the media, fans, and even other NFL players as a "very
physical team." As anyone who watches the sport for ten
minutes knows, football is a physical game. So, wouldn't it
stand to reason that we were a physical team? Were the
Cowboys or the Giants *unphysical* teams? Was that supposed to be a euphemism for wimpy? Or was being called
physical—which began as another cliché fostered by lazy
commentators because they couldn't come up with anything more specifically descriptive—a sanitized way of
saying "dirty"?

Many people considered Jack Tatum of the old Oakland
Raiders a dirty player. But even though the Steelers and the
Raiders had a tremendously "energetic" rivalry, I never felt
that he was anything but a hard-nosed, hard-hitting player.
Nor do I believe that Jack Tatum really intended to hurt
Darryl Stingley when he gave him that vicious hit during an
exhibition game; the collision unfortunately paralyzed
Stingley permanently. It was one of those tragic accidents
that happen in football.

Tatum had a reputation as a headhunter, but I think he
was taught to hit that way by his coaches. Later in his
career, when he played for the Oilers, Jack and I had an
especially memorable run-in at Three Rivers Stadium in

Pittsburgh. He had just written a book, *They Call Me Assassin*, in which he took a few cheap shots at Franco Harris, among others. Our fans were really after his scalp that day.

During the course of the game, Tatum briefly quieted the crowd when he intercepted a pass and took off down the sidelines. I hadn't even seen who made the interception; I just went after the white-and-blue jersey. I was really motoring toward this guy at a perfect angle, measuring him for a juicy hit. The last couple of yards, I fired up the afterburners and popped him full force at full-tilt speed. WHACK! I slammed into him at almost a ninety-degree angle, and he never knew what or who hit him. He landed on his head five yards out of bounds.

It was the hardest I'd ever hit anyone in football on any level, and it rocked the stadium. As he lay on the ground, I noticed it was our old friend Jack. I figured he'd be down for a while and was surprised when he was even able to get up. When he did, though, Tatum threw the ball in my face. I just looked at him and laughed.

"That's a fair trade," I said.

That was probably the longest conversation I'd had with an opposing player that season. As I've mentioned, the only real talking I did was with my teammates, especially the guys on the offensive line.

Communication was essential for us. We had to let each other know where we'd be or what we might be expecting. In the Steelers' offensive scheme, we had a lot of combination blocks—mostly double-teams—so there was a particular need for dialogue in order to move and execute in concert.

On the field, I did much of my chatting with two of the finest offensive linemen ever to play for the Steelers, Larry Brown and Mike Webster. For several years these two guys flanked me on the line—Bubba Brown on my right at tackle, Webbie on my left at center.

Let's say there was a defensive end lined up over Bubba and a defensive tackle over me, the right guard. On some routes, they'd loop around, with the charging end looking to make his turn and come straight over my ass to pop the quarterback. Our job was to stuff both of them, mainly using our hands (which is why we needed all that bench-press strength).

On this kind of play—which is called a loop stunt—I'd jam my hands straight out, *pa-boom*, and slam back my guy's shoulder pads. Then I'd hand him to Larry, slide back, and wait for the end to come steaming around. It was a very delicate and difficult maneuver (called an "area"—versus a man-to-man—block), like a well-choreographed, very violent dance. A mistimed step or slide and your buddy on the line is on his behind, soon to be followed by the glamorboy quarterback you've been paid such good money to protect.

After the game, I'd ask Larry back in the huddle: "Did you get that pass off okay, partner? Were you all right on that?" And Bubba would say, "Yeah, perfect," or—since he wasn't much of a talker on the field—just nod. Occasionally, he might suggest I try a different tack on my guy: "Next time, let's man it [go to a man-to-man block]."

For the most part, game action occurred too quickly for us to yell out, say "Switch!" in the middle of a play. Therefore, we had to plan for any contingency in the huddle. Knowing what our linemates would do, or where they'd be, would prevent most major surprises—and, on the offensive line, we *hated* surprises. So, these little tête-a-têtes in the huddle could literally save our buddy's ass—or his knee, leg, shoulder, etc.—from harm.

Or let's say there was a running play, a sweep left, with the noseguard lined up over Mike Webster and a linebacker in my face. We needed to do a seal combo—a combination block with Webbie and me sealing off the gap. But what if the noseguard looped around? If he looped left, Webbie would cut him off, and I'd sweep up on the linebacker. But if the nose came to me, I'd have to take him one on one, and Webbie would sweep up on the backer.

The whole thing was predicated on using the right footwork—you had to step a certain way—in addition to planning and communication. A lot of times on double-team or read blocks, we talked tactics in the huddle regarding hand placements or splits, doing whatever we could to help each other out.

A smart defensive coach will try and confuse offenses with many different looks, and will often change the attack right before the snap. In a blink, the offensive lineman has to be ready for all those looks and sets, and has to react immediately to every possibility. Because of these split-second reactions, I have never encountered a stupid offensive lineman. (I can't say the same for the other positions, however.) I've known some who were more erudite or learned than others, but all were instinctively intelligent men.

It was also of great importance that these bright, communicative men remain in control of their tempers at all times. We couldn't have one guy getting so pissed at his man that he'd freelance and try to run him down. We needed him to be where we expected him to be. With the exception of quarterback, no other position on the field requires as much discipline and patience. Unlike the QB, however, we had to be willing at all times to sublimate our ego, as well as our anger, for the good of the team. (Our line coach, Rollie Dotsch, would constantly remind us: "Stay cool, controlled and calculated." It was like our mantra.)

On the offensive line, you simply cannot just tee off on people; you need to adhere to a well-defined scheme. Defensive linemen can paw at the ground like bulls and charge at you with everything they've got, but an offensive lineman has to stand and fight. Whatever aggression is utilized, again, must be *controlled.*

Obviously, it's the job of the defensive players and coaches to try and rattle the offense—to take the linemen, in particular, out of their game and as far away as possible from being in control. Two defensive coordinators stand out in that regard–Hank Bullough of the Bengals and the Bears' Buddy Ryan. Buddy was a master motivator, a real players' coach, as well as a tactical innovator; he would go to the mat against management if he felt his players were being mistreated (that quality likely got him fired from his subsequent job as head coach of the Eagles), and his players would run through walls (and offensive linemen) for him.

Bullough was more a master of strategy; he invariably installed more defensive sets than any other team. In a game with Cincinnati, we might be faced with a look (defensive positioning) that had never before been seen in the NFL. He would move outside linebacker Reggie Williams all over the field; on any given play, we never knew where Reggie was going to line up.

This was an added challenge to Rollie Dotsch since he and Hank were such good friends. They would derive special pleasure from beating the other guy. When there's talk about the game within a game, it usually refers to player matchups. When the Bengals played the Steelers, one of the key rivalries was Hank versus Rollie. Often the man who came up with *the* innovative tactical maneuver was the one who helped win the war.

The most memorable matchups I had were one-on-one, mano-à-mano, head-to-head-banging, trench-shaking situations where, for most of the game, it was my strength, technique, and controlled aggression against a defensive lineman's strength, speed, and untrammeled fury. I was always more jazzed up when I went up against great players such as Randy White, Dan Hampton, Howie Long, Curley Culp, and Bob Golic, who personified all of those exceptional traits.

Curley was a real handful because he was not that tall. I always felt that squat, beefy offensive linemen had an advantage over rangy defensive linemen because we could get under those skyscrapers' shoulder pads with a little extra leverage. Golic was another guy who wasn't that big, but who used his wrestling skills to maneuver out of double-team predicaments.

For some reason, toward the end of my career in Tampa Bay I had the most trouble with Doug English of the Detroit Lions. He may not have been as physically gifted as some of those other guys, but he was a master technician at countering moves. For one, he knew that if I got my hands on him, I could use sheer strength to steer him one way or another. So he would always try and slap my hands away, never letting me get any leverage on him. He didn't try to play a power game, which many linemen often did. I could usually handle the brutes who wanted to match me strength for strength; it was the tactical players who gave me the most difficulty.

Doug was also a class guy. I remember one game in which we were about to run out the clock with a small lead, and Doug and his teammates were ordered to attack full bore on the final play. Most times, after the snap is made, the quarterback falls to his knees and the defense just taps him gently on the pads or helmet—as much a gesture of concession as any real effort. On this day, for some strange reason, the coach had demanded that his players go all out on the last play. Fortunately, Doug and most of his teammates chose not to follow this absurd order (which no doubt made for some interesting postgame discussions in the Lions' lockerroom).

During games, most coaches work off their frustrations by screaming at players. Most of the time, you don't really pay much attention. As a young player trying to impress, however, you find yourself conscious of every cutting remark, as well as every pat on the back. Most rookies don't have the built-in confidence to ignore the opinions and whims of their coaches; and, of course, it is the coaches themselves, who are responsible for this climate of uncertainty and insecurity. As long as the player is off-balance, the power lies with the coach. He determines how a player feels about himself and as such, can more easily manipulate an inexperienced player. A centered, confident player knows what he can do on the field (and what he can get away with off of it).

As a young player eager to please, I'd jump every time my coaches kicked or screamed. As an inexperienced player, in '79, I was having some trouble with the seemingly complicated defensive schemes of the St. Louis Cardinals. Early in the game, I misread a blitz and Bradshaw got stomped; he was taken out of the game with what looked like a broken ankle. I knew it was my fault, and I felt like crap. George Perles, the defensive coach, seconded that notion. He kept jumping up and down, yelling at me from the sidelines that I was a "no-good pile o' fleashit."

I felt humiliated enough and did not need anyone else piling on. Fortunately, Brad—who never said a discouraging or negative word to me then or since—came back in the second half and led us to an exciting, come-from-behind win. My gaffe was mercifully forgotten until the Tuesday film critique.

Needless to say, the worse moment for an offensive lineman is when you give up a sack and your quarterback goes down hard. You could stuff your guy the whole game, just dominate him from end to end, but if he gets around you for one freaking sack, he's dancing up and down like his team just won the Super Bowl. Like all offensive linemen, I never cared much for those histrionic displays.

By the way, when's the last time you saw an offensive lineman whoop it up and dance around? How would it look if we did a little cha-cha every time our opponent did *not* reach the quarterback?

The offensive lineman just does his job. Unfortunately, the average fan only notices him when he screws up. You can imagine how delighted we were when the NFL decided to have its officials announce to the stadium and television audience the identity of all penalty perpetrators, since the most common foul called is that of offensive holding. Think about it: the only time an offensive lineman's number is called is when it's for some infraction.

You can't play on the offensive line and be a glory hound. You must accept that fans won't ever scream your name in ecstasy unless you fall on a fumble or, God love us, return one for a touchdown. The times you usually hear it from the crowd are when they're screaming for your scalp. You must have a thick skin and a strong sense of self. That's one of the key reasons why so many successful coaches began their careers on the offensive line. Look over there on the Steeler sideline, and you'll still see one.

Self-sacrifice is the cornerstone of an offensive lineman's professional life. You're on the low end of the pay scale. You're required to play with more injuries. You're responsible for the well-being of the so-called "skill" positions, particularly quarterback and running back. And you're expected to train harder and longer than anyone on the team.

You may see a linebacker drop into the weight room now and then, some running backs, even a quarterback (but only if he's rehabilitating from an injury). But without question, with or without chemical assistance, the offensive line has always spent more time in the weight room than any other group of football players.

For us, the battle is never over.

My most memorable battle was Super Bowl XIII against the Cowboys in 1979, the only one I played in. (The following year, in Super Bowl XIV, I was hurt and couldn't play.)

The feeling I had walking out on field at the Orange Bowl in Miami was that of intensity and also one of airiness, if that's the right word—tight and light at the same time. My stomach was tight from nerves, blood steaming with adrenaline, while my head and body felt so light that my feet seemed to be propelled by a cushion of air.

The fear of failure was the most overwhelming I had ever seen. No one wanted to be the guy who cost his team the game. That's why most of the Super Bowl games have been either one-sided blowouts or very conservative, boring affairs. Each mistake is magnified a hundredfold. Look at Jackie Smith, who, in this very game, dropped the ball in the end zone for what would have been the Cowboys' winning score, and had to live with the shame and ignominy for the rest of his life.

You didn't want to let yourself down, and you certainly didn't want to let your teammates down. If you had a good year, you especially didn't want to spoil it with a lackluster performance in the BIGGEST GAME OF YOUR LIFE. And yes, you do think in those hyperbolic terms.

This was *it*. This was what you had worked for since training camp, what you had probably imagined since you were 10 or 12 years old ("10 seconds left in the game . . . there's Courson off tackle going in for the winning score . . . the gun sounds as his teammates carry him off the field to the deafening cheers of the crowd . . .").

In fact, your football life does sort of flash before you, with memories of pee-wee, high school, college, and even some of your earlier games in the pros. But the collective pressure of all those contests does not even begin to approach the intensity and hype of this one game.

The Steelers were particularly fired up at the start, whacking shoulder pads and even helmets and yelling encouragement—much of it profane—at one another. Usually we went about jobs in a more professional and businesslike manner, but the team was going for its third Super Bowl in five years—something no other franchise had accomplished—and there was a deeper sense of mission that day.

I was in on the opening kickoff, with Dallas receiving, the only offensive lineman on this special team because of my speed. Basically my job was go to the edge of the wedge and turn the play inside. I was called the Hash Man, not an enviable job—particularly with the chop block still in the game.

I remember looking up at the sky and thinking how unusual that it would be so gray in Miami. The clouds were dark, threatening. The sound, of course, was deafening. I had heard noise like this before—our fans were among the most loyal and vocal in the league—but it seemed that every one of the 80,000 or so fans in the stadium were unleashing the full fury of their lungs and vocal chords. And yet I was strangely calm and even detached in the proverbial eye of the storm. I actually *felt* the noise more than I heard it.

Once the game began and we took our first hits, the players seemed to relax. I think it was the coaches on both sides who remained tight. It was a hell of a game, probably the most exciting Super Bowl up until then, with plenty of scoring and a near-miraculous comeback by Dallas. We held on to win, 35–31, though if Jackie Smith had controlled that ball in his breadbasket, the Cowboys likely would have won and the Steelers wouldn't have put on their third Super Bowl ring. Ultimately, it came down to mistakes. We made a few; Dallas made more.

Bradshaw played inspired football. It was one of those days that you could tell on the sidelines. He had the *look*—a look of such intensity, confidence, and mastery that the rest of us knew that if we just did our jobs, we would win. I imagine the feeling to be similar to the confidence that great generals inspire on the day of their biggest battles. The troops sense that their leader is in complete control and just wait for their orders.

Unfortunately for us, Roger Staubach was in control too. Prior to the game, the guy who scared us the most was Tony Dorsett—he was the league's leading breakaway threat—and we keyed on him much of the game. Though he did get loose a couple of times, breaking a tackle trap early for a long gain, he was never a real factor. As it turned out, Drew Pearson and Tony Hill became the main weapons in Staubach's arsenal.

I didn't play that much, mostly special teams and some key third-down situations. I didn't make any tackles on kickoffs, but I didn't make any mistakes either—no holding penalties. My greatest regret was that I didn't recover a fumble on a kickoff. The ball had squibbed loose on a short kick to the Cowboys' defensive end Randy White, and for a moment I had it in my hands. But I couldn't hold on. Fortunately—again, for us—Tony Dungy recovered it, and we marched in for a score.

For years thereafter, I'd replay that fumble in my mind—my little shot at football immortality. I even dreamt about it. But time and again, the ball slipped through my fingers.

I was 24 years old. (Had I not gotten injured the following

year, I would have been the youngest starter, next to cornerback Ron Johnson, to play in Super Bowl XIV.) I assumed then that there would be plenty of other opportunities for greater glory later in my career.

That assumption would prove to be false.

5

PLAYERS AND COACHING

I PLAYED FOR seven years on one of the most storied teams in all of sports, the Pittsburgh Steelers: four Super Bowl wins in six years ('75, '76, '79, '80). Six players (Bradshaw, Greene, Harris, Lambert, Ham, Blount) are already in the Hall of Fame; and three or four more (Webster, Stallworth, Swann, Greenwood) and one coach (Noll) are likely to be inducted.

When fans find out I was a Steeler during a good part of those glory years—some folks remember me, some don't— they want to know what Bradshaw or Noll or Lambert were really like. Occasionally sportscasters or sportswriters will ask me to free-associate about my ex-teammates and coaches. So, off the top of my head (with only minimal rewriting—or rethinking), here are some thumbnail sketches of several men whom I played with and for on the Pittsburgh Steelers, in additional to some thoughts on the state of coaching in the NFL and elsewhere.

THE PLAYERS (OFFENSE)

MATT BAHR (STEELERS, 1979–80): Kickers are rarely accepted as an integral part of a football team; they're usually perceived as flaky, wimpy midgets who frequently find themselves with the fate of the team in their feet. On the Steelers, we actually liked Matt. He was a congenial, easy-going, intelligent kid who just did his job. And because of our affection for him, we would often make him the butt of our pranks—the cruelest of which was when six of us taped him into the laundry cart, poured shaving cream all over him, and left the cart sitting for 10 minutes in Chuck Noll's office.

Matt, who was a good sport about it (like he had much of a choice) later told us that Old Stoneface shook his head and actually sort of half-smiled when he found the kicker in his office. I was very happy for Matt's success with the Giants leading up to (and in) the team's 1991 Super Bowl victory.

ROCKY BLEIER (STEELERS, 1971–80): Nothing and nobody intimidated the Rock. Considering the harrowing real-life dangers and wounds he experienced in Vietnam, the simulated warfare of professional football was a piece of cake for him. Basically quiet and even shy in the clubhouse, he led more by example. So, I'm a little surprised that he's become such an accomplished motivational speaker and broadcaster. As such, he's a lot smoother and more polished than the working-class type I remember.

Some running backs on the Steelers used steroids, but the Rock is the only one who's on record. He says that he took steroids primarily as a recuperative device to overcome a shrapnel injury in his leg incurred in Vietnam. He was also one of the few running backs I played with who spent a lot of time in the weight room.

TERRY BRADSHAW (STEELERS, 1970–82): I've already given my take on Brad in Chapter 2. As I said, I liked and respected him greatly, but never really got to know him. I wish I had. An awesome talent with an "aw-shucks" style, he had a great arm, size, mobility, toughness, and, viewers can hear on his NFL broadcasts, intelligence. I think Brad also might have been hypersensitive, which might have made it difficult for him to deal with the demands of the fans and, particularly, his head coach. There wouldn't have been any Super Bowl rings for the Pittsburgh Steelers—much less four—without Terry Bradshaw.

When he first became a broadcaster for CBS, I was playing down in Tampa. Whenever Brad came down there to do a game, he was very conscious of how unhappy I was with the Bucs and went out of his way to encourage me. I always appreciated that.

FRANCO HARRIS (STEELERS, 1972–83): A true Hall of Famer and, contrary to some folks' opinion, a real gamer.

There's been talk over the years that some of the Steelers may have resented our star runner. Jim Brown, among others, has criticized Franco for running out of bounds, for not taking the extra yard, for not taking the hits. Brown was a great running back—maybe the best ever—but he's out of his league when he denigrates Franco.

Franco was well liked in the locker room, and always kept the guys loose with an encouraging comment or a wisecrack. And he could take it as well as dish it out.

The offensive line had a nickname for Franco: Sting Bee. This had to do with his inability or, shall we say, his unwillingness to block. Before each game, we'd pass Franco's locker and say, "Hey, Bee, you gonna sting 'em today?" And Franco, who knew we were kidding about his blocking, would just nod and laugh. "Yep, guys, I'm gonna sting 'em big time."

With the game on the line, though, Franco could block as well as anyone. And we knew he'd be there when it counted. He was one of the great money players of his era.

Franco was very smart. He knew that running backs who got hurt or who got hit a lot weren't going to last long in the NFL. The backs who tried for that extra yard when they were being stood up in the pile were the ones likely to be injured. There's a fine line between macho and stupidity. Most of us liked and respected Franco too much to begrudge him that extra yard not taken.

THE CHINA DOLLS—JOHN STALLWORTH (STEELERS, 1974–87) AND LYNN SWANN (STEELERS, 1974–82): A couple of other guys who were there when we needed them were the receivers we called our China Dolls, Swann and Stallworth. The coaches would tell us in practice: "Don't hit the wide receivers." Hell, we got smacked around pretty good, but I don't remember hearing, "Don't hit the offensive lineman."

The fact that we liked our two little China Dolls tremendously only increased our ribbing of their "delicate" constitutions. We knew that if Swannie had to go over the middle only one time during a game, he'd make the catch, take the hit, and never say a word. And we also knew that Stall, whose career may have been overshadowed by Swannie's more flamboyant circus act, was the most consistent, persistent receiver the Steelers ever had.

John didn't talk much, and led by quiet example. Swannie, you couldn't get him to shut his mouth—either from talking or smiling. I'd sometimes get pissed off because the guy was always in a good mood. It didn't matter if it was exhibition practice or a Super Bowl; he invariably seemed to be having a great time. It's no surprise that he's parlayed that extroverted nature into a nice little show biz career; recently, he was the host of a game show, "To Tell the Truth." And if truth be told, he wasn't half bad.

As football players, Stall had a little more speed, but Swannie's soft hands and acrobatic abilities were unmatched. Because of his career stats, Stall might be a more likely Hall of Fame choice, but my bet is both will make it.

LARRY BROWN (STEELERS, 1971–84): Bubba (a.k.a. the Boss) Brown and John Kolb were the best tackle tandem in the league. At right tackle, Bubba ran the show on the offensive line because . . . well, because he was the Boss. He was especially effective as a pass blocker. I've seen him dominate his opponent so thoroughly for two quarters that the guy would virtually quit in the second half. In viewing the game films afterward, we'd sit in awe and softly chant: "Boss . . . Boss . . . Boss." To observe a 280-pound black man blush was quite a sight.

Bubba was another weight-room junkie, I once saw him bench 500 pounds with a close (12 inches apart) grip. Knee problems prevented Bubba from being as good a drive blocker as he could have been, but the fact that he only made the Pro Bowl once was a crime. His retirement after 14 years added to the longevity of several defensive linemen in the league.

SAM DAVIS (STEELERS, 1967–79): Befitting his stature as grand old man on the Steeler line, Davis picked up the nickname Riggy (for rigor mortis). He was the coolest, steadiest guy in pressure situations, and would help keep the rest of us calm. Ironically, his other nickname was the Tight Man, reputedly because he'd get so anxious during film sessions, like an actor who hated to watch himself.

Sam was also one of the more compassionate men I've met in the game. Whenever anyone got injured, he'd take the time to empathize and encourage the player (too often, a disabled player is treated like a leper, as if the injury is contagious). Riggy always knew the right thing to say. A natural leader and one-time Steeler captain, he was the classic pulling guard—quick, smart, undersized—before steroids and weights built bigger specimens.

TUNCH ILKIN (STEELERS, 1980–PRESENT): Born in Istanbul (his mom was Miss Turkey in the fifties), he's lasted more than a decade on the team that originally cut him. In 1980, Tunch was a victim of a numbers game on the Steelers—too many good offensive linemen—and he was devastated by his misfortune. But when I was put on injured reserve with a dislocated foot, he quit his job at a health club to return to the Steelers. We immediately became good friends.

Probably the smallest offensive tackle in the NFL today, the Mad Turk is a fanatical weightlifter and martial arts aficionado. Back in our wild youth, the Tuncher was one of our key running mates. During the Urban Cowboy craze of 1980, every bar had a mechanical bull, and at this one place in suburban Pittsburgh, Tunch made it his mission to beat that bull. For hours, he tried to ride that thing—he kept getting thrown, but he kept getting back on—until he looked like a 250-pound rag doll. Though he never really beat it, he never gave up . . . and that's Tunch. A great leader and a great competitor.

JON KOLB (STEELERS, 1969–81): Along with Webster and me, Kolbie spent more time in the weight room than any other Steeler (which, in those days, meant more than any other NFL player); he was one of the strongest men ever to play the game. A quiet guy with a fierce desire to succeed, Jon utilized his God-given abilities as much as anyone I've seen.

Toward the end of his career, nagging injuries slowed him down, but he remained a clubhouse leader. I didn't think Kolbie would end up as a coach (particularly with the Steelers, since he didn't seem to be that fond of Chuck)—

initially of the defensive line, and now as the strength coach. The latter is his real forte; Kolbie knows as much about strength technique as anyone in the NFL. When he competed in the World's Strongest Man Competition, against élite weightlifters (often giving away 60 or 70 pounds), he'd always come back with some great training tips.

Kolbie is originally from Oklahoma, and I thought he'd return to his farm in Washington County, south of Pittsburgh. I never figured he had the temperament, or the inclination, to play the political games necessary for NFL coaches.

GERRY MULLINS (STEELERS, 1971–79): "Moon" was a fun-loving bachelor who always had pretty women chasing after him when I lived with him on the North Side my second year. I was his understudy on and off the football field. Sort of a philosophizer-rogue, Moon was a realist who never let himself get caught up in the rah-rah bullshit of Steeler football.

Moon was one of the smallest guards in the NFL at the time, which is why he became such a skilled technician. My rookie season, one of the Steeler assistant coaches gave Moon some Dianabol to put on some poundage (he had lost even more weight from his "light" frame due to the flu). Moon threw the pills away.

A great athlete who had played tight end at U.S.C. with O. J. Simpson, he was occasionally utilized in that capacity by the Steelers, mainly on short-yardage situations. Moon was always an avid outdoorsman—we called him the Great White Hunter—and I'm surprised he's stayed in the Pittsburgh area (I think to be close to his young son). He now works for a metal and minerals distributor.

TED PETERSEN (STEELERS, 1977–83): Pete and I broke into the league together in '77. Tall and lean, he would've been very scary had he gone chemical. As it was, after a couple of years playing behind Bubba and Kolbie, he became a very solid offensive tackle.

Extremely soft-spoken and gentle off the field, you wonder how he ever manufactured the necessary fire for football; yet I remember a few times when Petey would get downright mean and even come out swinging (usually on special teams after a cheap shot).

Pete is now doing what I always thought he'd be good at: coaching kids. A very patient, intelligent, and congenial man, he's also my boss (I'm one of his assistants at Trinity High School in Washington, 30 miles southwest of Pittsburgh).

RAY PINNEY (STEELERS, 1976–78, 1980–82): Another blocking machine at utility lineman (originally drafted by the Steelers as a center, he played mostly offensive tackle and some guard). We called him the Rubber Man because he could recover so quickly from a precarious position and still dominate the block.

He left the Steelers to play for a couple of years in the USFL for the Michigan Panthers, but, uncharacteristically for Chuck Noll, was welcomed back with open arms when that upstart league folded.

MIKE WEBSTER (STEELERS, 1974–88): Nine Pro Bowls, four Super Bowl wins, Steeler team captain, a lock as a Hall of Famer; the greatest center ever to play in the NFL, one of the greatest offensive linemen of all time, and one of my closest friends. He is also one of the most intelligent, caring, and honest people I know. And the hardest worker.

My rookie year, the older veterans used to haze him a bit about being so relentless and "gung-ho" about football. "Webbie," they said, "you'll be here forever." In the NFL, 17 years *is* forever, and that's how long he lasted (until his retirement last year from the Kansas City Chiefs). In all that time, he played every down as if it was his last. In fact, from the beginning of the 1976 season until the playoff game against the San Diego in 1982, in which he turned his ankle, Webbie took every snap in every game.

Out of football now for only a year, Webbie has even more to give off the field. Recently hired as an analyst on NBC football telecasts, he'll no doubt put the same energy and effort into that arena as he did to his magnificent athletic career.

When I was diagnosed with heart disease, Mike Webster came through in spades. An unassuming, humble man, he offered to sponsor a roast in his honor—and donated the bulk of the proceeds to a medical trust fund that had been set up for my health care (any overages in the fund will go to needy people).

For my money, he's simply the best.

DEFENSE

MEL BLOUNT (STEELERS, 1970–83):   The prototypical cornerback of his day. Great cover guy, nasty hitter, respected leader. Married through most of his career, he never hung out much with the guys (or at least the guys in my gang); therefore, I didn't get to know him as well as I would've liked.

"Supe" is as much an asset to the community today as he was to the great Steeler teams. His work with the Mel Blount Youth Home, just south of Pittsburgh, is typical of the selfless, dedicated manner in which he's conducted all aspects of his personal and professional life.

GARY DUNN (STEELERS, 1977–87):   If the number of nicknames a fellow has is any indication of the esteem in which he is held by his compatriots, Dunnie—a.k.a. Nuke, Disco, Fat

Albert, His Fatness—was easily the best-loved player on the Steelers (Nuke for being the nucleus of the defense, His Fatness for more obvious reasons). A big bear with a huge heart, he'd bust your chops at every opportunity.

We had a lot in common: about the same age, single, we both liked to go out and raised a little hell, maybe even lift a few skirts. Some folks couldn't deal with our fun; because of our sheer size and exuberance, they were often afraid that we'd start busting up furniture and people. But we never looked to take out our aggressions on anybody else (mailboxes and stop signs notwithstanding). We just liked to drink a few beers and howl at the moon.

Because he wasn't a "bonus baby"—in addition to following in Joe Greene's massive footsteps—Gary was an underrated player. But he was smart, strong, industrious, quick as a panther, and ultimately enjoyed a long, productive career.

Dunnie's living down in the Florida Keys now, trying to find the key to the second half of his life. We still speak every few weeks on the phone. He recently took a job with Budweiser. But now, with access to the company product, Dunnie told me: "I don't know if it's a good or a bad thing. Ten years ago, I would've appreciated [the unlimited beer] more."

JOE GREENE (STEELERS, 1969–81):   I had heard stories and seen films of the "Mean Joe" Greene who would sooner kick you when you were down than help you up. (In his rookie year, he spat in a reporter's face.) But I only played with "Gentleman Joe," a thoroughly intelligent, relentless, focused, and dignified professional who was the heart of the Steeler team.

For some reason he took an interest in me early on. On the last day of practice in 1977, my first year with the Steelers, we were in the dressing room packing up to go to Denver. And Joe came over to shake my hand. He knew I was disheartened, having spent the entire year on injured reserve—which meant I could play with the team in practice, but not on game days. I was wondering what kind of future, if any, I had in football. Joe thanked me for sticking it out all season, and for working so hard.

"You're going to be a player in this league," he said to me. Then he gave me a few tips on how I could prepare in the off-season. The fact that Joe Greene would take the time to pat me on the back, to thank *me*, was truly overwhelming. And it gave me an enormous incentive to come back and play up to my potential.

Several years later, Joe was reminded of that encounter. In response, he said: "All I told [Steve] was to go into the off-season with the idea of not wasting it. . . . The coaches knew he had a future here. The team knew it. And I knew it."

I may have returned the favor in a small way by helping to motivate Joe with weight training. Throughout most of his career, he was just a tremendously big, strong, quick athlete who allowed his natural ability to carry him to great success. But in practice he was playing against weight-room junkies like myself and Mike Webster. And in his latter football years, seeing how the work was paying off for us, he started to train more with weights. Joe later admitted that it helped prolong his career, and even helped him to play better. (I hear Lawrence Taylor of the Giants was similar in this regard; past 30, he finally began a real training regimen).

Joe's currently the defensive line coach at Pittsburgh.

L. C. GREENWOOD (STEELERS, 1969–81): On a team loaded with characters, Hollywood Bags was an original. He was a constant source of humor in the locker room. Extremely observant—and sarcastic—he was the first to observe anyone's failings or physical oddities, and equally quick with a cutting comment. Emanating from the right corner of the locker room (where his locker was located) was a running stream of commentary, usually accompanied by that low, slow, infectious laugh.

Tall, strong, and fast, Bags probably would have made a great power forward in the NBA. But, then again, he wouldn't have had as much opportunity to hit people. Bags had a great attitude about football: it was *only* a game, and he was there to have fun. One of the quickest defensive linemen in the game, Bags loved to juke and improvise, giving his opponent across the line absolute fits. It's amazing how he remained such a productive football player for so long considering he was positively allergic to the weight room. The only time I remember him in there was to make fun of the rest of us.

JACK HAM (STEELERS, 1971–82): Not too big, not too fast, yet a tremendously hard-nosed player with great athletic talents. The best pass-covering linebacker of his era. He was probably underrated at the time because he was so solid and consistent, never loud or flashy. Hammer didn't spend much time in the weight room, but he had an instinctive knack for the game. I don't recall ever seeing him out of position.

A very intelligent player, Jack has done well in his business interests in the Pittsburgh area; he's also done some local announcing work. Hammer is still close to the Rooneys and Chuck, so you'll never hear a discouraging word from him about the Steeler organization.

JACK LAMBERT (STEELERS, 1974–84): I've spoken at some length about Jack, and while we may not be the most compatible of men, that doesn't diminish the respect I had for Jack as a football player. If Joe Greene was the heart of the Steelers, Jack was the soul. He was the personification of Pittsburgh's hard-working, in-your-face, shot-and-a-beer mentality.

Only 230 pounds, Lammy was the most dominant middle linebacker of his day, and a worthy heir to Huff, Nitschke, and Butkus. He did it on talent, guts, intelligence, and extraordinary energy. Probably the most intense guys I've encountered in civilian life. I often think that Jack is still trapped by that surly, snarling image. For his sake, I hope he has slowed down and begun to enjoy life more.

THE COACHES

ROLLIE DOTSCH: My favorite and most respected line coach. He knew his players as well as he knew X's and O's, an exception to most coaches who never played in the NFL. Rollie was also not the typical heartless coach who only cared about winning; he had compassion for the men who were playing hurt, and never pushed us beyond our limits. He would even party with us on occasion. At one postseason blowout, some of the young players challenged me to a drinking contest—double shots of kamikazes. Rollie said he'd also like to participate. So we're all downing three, four, five shots before the younger players start falling out—or down. But Rollie's keeping up; he seems barely buzzed. Then someone discovers he's chugging shots of water.

Rollie died in 1988 from cancer. When I saw him for the last time, a month before he succumbed, he had lost more than 50 pounds. I was glad that I could tell him face to face how much he had meant to me, and how much I valued playing for him. I miss him greatly.

BILL MEYERS: Not one of my favorite coaches. A former Marine, he mistook screaming and yelling for teaching. During my last year with the Steelers, he minimized the severity of my knee problems and was probably instrumental in me being traded to Tampa Bay.

Though we had our differences, Bill showed some class when he came to a benefit for me in March 1991—a charity basketball game between former Steelers and local radio personalities. We had a nice chat and discovered that both of us have probably mellowed over the years.

DAN RADAKOVICH: My first line coach with the Steelers, he liked to live up to the nickname of "Bad Rad." While I felt that his abrasive, manipulative methods were unnecessary and contrived—he loved to screw with our minds—I thought he was a technical genius. Often credited with introducing the "punch" move in pass blocking, he also refined many of the now-accepted techniques on hand placement and footwork.

I remember Rad storming into our meeting room one day, holding up a copy of Jerry Sandusky's book, *Penn State Linebacking*. "This guy plagiarized my mind!" he shouted. Before coming to the Steelers, Rad had been the linebacker coach for Joe Paterno at State and felt (possibly rightly) that he was the motivating force behind all those great backers. He ranted and raved about this for days.

CHUCK NOLL: Terry Bradshaw devoted a 20-page chapter in his book to Chuck. In sheer word count, I've probably doubled that output. Like Brad, I have thoroughly ambivalent feelings about my former head coach. I'm grateful to him for having given me the opportunity to play with the Steelers; yet I'm still disappointed and (though I hate to admit it) bitter about the way he callously discarded me from the team.

Chuck Noll is, in many ways, a brilliant man; he understands the technical aspects of the game as well as anyone. Yet he's stubborn and rigid, and often refuses to adapt to the changing face of football. He wouldn't even use the shotgun formation until about two years ago.

His psychological bag of tricks is equally outmoded. What worked for us Neanderthals 15 years ago does not play today. The only constant seems to be his players' universal dislike for him. Chuck has never been a player's coach.

Myron Cope, the longtime voice of the Steelers and the man behind the Terrible Towel craze, once dubbed Chuck the "Emperor Chas." It was probably as much a statement about Chuck's imperious manner as it was of his success. My feeling is that, for the most part, this emperor has no clothes. The people of Pittsburgh don't really want to acknowledge or accept that fact. They prefer to look at him as their hero. Chuck Noll is obviously a very competent football coach, but I don't think he should be anybody's hero.

I have never heard one word—encouraging or otherwise—from Chuck Noll since I left the Steelers. When my heart illness was publicized, virtually everyone connected to the team contacted me or made some gesture of support. Not Chuck. It was as if I ceased to exist once I departed from the Steelers. This from a man who preached time and again about team loyalty.

Why are athletes so naïve? Are we such needy children that we can be so easily fooled by the "tough but fair" talk of these phony father figures? I don't understand why it takes so long for us to figure out that the talk and the men are hollow. We should be able to see that the coach's need for us is temporary. Let's face it: All they really want to know is, "What can you do for me *now*?"

And as soon as your "now" is past, you're history.

Most coaches are like Chuck Noll because most coaches want to be like Chuck Noll. Or Tom Landry, Joe Gibbs, or Bill Parcells. Or the legendary Vince Lombardi. Winning soon becomes the only thing. And in order to become successful coaches, would-be legends mistakenly believe that the only way to get their team's respect is fear—often created with inhumane, abusive treatment. They're not man enough to treat their players like men.

Presumably men can take care of themselves. But what about the kids? Too often you see a pee-wee player or a Little Leaguer make a mistake, and the coach quickly jumps all over the poor kid.

"Don't do that!" the coach yells.

Instead of harping on what the kid should not do, the coach should be enthusiastically telling the kid what he (or she) *can* do. A coach cannot positively reinforce a kid too much.

Most pee-wee coaches are just parents who don't know any better. But what about the so-called professionals, the high school and small-college coaches who aspire to something greater? They, too, should know better.

In high school, I was lucky. I had a coach who recognized that his players were young men, big boys even, who didn't want or need to be lied to, manipulated, or threatened. He just coached us.

When I went to college, I was told (and fell for) some of the Big Lies that coaches on that level have been spreading for years. They were (and are): 1) You will play big-time college football; 2) you will enjoy playing big-time college football; 3) you will be drafted by the NFL; 4) then you will have a long and successful career in the NFL; 5) throughout your pro career, you will be surrounded by people who are truly interested in you; 6) after your retirement, your NFL coach will maintain an interest in you; 7) many benefits, financial and otherwise, will continue to accrue to you; and 8) you will live long enough to collect your NFL pension.

Not all college or pro coaches are lying, cheating, ego-driven opportunists. There are a few coaches in the NFL and in college who are worthy of respect. One of the coaches I admire a great deal is Joe Paterno, particularly on the steroid issue. After the controversy at Notre Dame when former player Steve Huffman accused coach Lou Holtz of knowing about the team's steroid use, Paterno said, that he couldn't be sure all his players were clean—as Holtz contended—but that they were going to do the best they could with testing; if anyone got caught, they'd be finished for the year. That's as honest as any Division I coach has been.

Paterno has always stressed education. Penn State is not some football factory, which has made it a tougher sell to some kids. When Paterno recruits an athlete, he sells the parents on the legitimately high graduation rate—not just P.E. courses, but real studies. That's smart coaching. No program is squeaky clean, but I do believe that Penn State is better than most.

I always wished that Paterno had recruited me. Maybe I could have become one of those legendary linebackers. Who knows? I might not ever have found a need to take steroids.

6

A TALE OF
TWO CITIES—
PITTSBURGH
AND TAMPA BAY

I PLAYED IN Pittsburgh during the height of Steeler mania. During this time—the mid-seventies through the early eighties—the team and the city were indistinguishable. The Steelers were as much a part of Pittsburgh's infrastructure as its roads or its three rivers, and politicians routinely invoked our name to claim a little glory as their own.

The relationship between the fans and players was extremely intense. It was intense on the field, and it was intense after the game, usually in celebration, at the local watering holes.

This being a boilermaker town, the offensive linemen were stars. The fans related to us; they appreciated our dusky, musky work. And while we never approached the celebrity and adulation of the Bradshaws, the Swanns, or the Lamberts, we were still mightily revered and respected. Everyone wanted to be our friends, to buy us a shot or two, a beer or three.

It was a magical time in a great city, and I never wanted to leave.

My final days as a Steeler were painful ones.

During the second half of the '83 season I played despite the pains in my knees. And then, after limping around much of the off-season, I spent hours and hours in the Nautilus rehab room trying to build up my quadriceps.

I went into training camp in 1984 mentally ready to go, but I soon found the physical discomfort as bad as anything I had ever experienced. I rarely mentioned my injuries to the coaching or training staff—I just tried to block them out and go about my business—but when I tried to go full out, there was great pain. I told the coaches and trainers that my knee was really screwed up, but they didn't seem to care much. They put me on anti-inflammatories (Celestone and Clinoril) and basically said that if I couldn't cut it, they'd bring in some young stud who could.

I was disheartened, discouraged, and dismayed. With the whole season in front of me, I was in agony. And worse, nobody gave a shit. It was right about then that I lost all the faith in the Steelers and their system.

Running drills, I felt as if my knee was going to blow at any time. I stormed off the practice field and into the locker room in frustration and disgust. I threw down my helmet so hard a piece of the face mask shattered. The trainer asked what was wrong.

"My knee's killing me," I said. "I can't run. I can't practice."

Chuck Noll was angry. Mostly he was annoyed that I had waited this long in camp to tell him that I couldn't practice. I should have said something earlier, he said. I was about to tell him that I *had* told the other coaches, but that nobody seemed to give a flying . . .

He cut me off; he didn't want to hear it. He was so furious that he was spitting on me as he screamed.

His anger toward me was entirely impersonal. It was like I was some stranger who had cut him off in the parking lot. There was not one iota of sympathy or concern on his part. He wasn't even addressing me as a human being, certainly not one who had worked so hard for him, who had played so hard for him, and who had achieved so much for him and for the team. My pain was irrelevant; his only concern was that I had spoiled his game plan.

Later, in our team meeting, he reamed me out in front of the team for my selfishness and lack of team spirit. He also fined me $100, just to break my balls a little more. Chuck had always liked to pick on me: I was a big target, and maybe he thought I could take it. The year before, he had singled me out after I pulled a hamstring, giving me all that crap about using steroids and bodybuilding.

After the meeting, I was incensed. I went up to him—right in his face—and said, "We need to talk."

I had had my fill of his psychological manipulations, his bullying, his coldness. I was angry, but I was also hurt. I wasn't just some big, dumb lapdog he could kick all over the field and who would come back panting for more. This dog already had his day.

By the time we finally talked behind closed doors, both of us had calmed down. On Chuck's part, he had no need to flay me further. The public flogging was done as much for the rookies as for me. ("Jeez," they're supposed to think, "if this is how he treats a seven-year veteran, a guy who's been to the Pro Bowl and two Super Bowls, we better not get out of line.") Chuck may have been calm, but he was still patronizing—telling me that I needed to practice technique and drills.

"You need the work," he said.

"After seven years," I said, "how much more are you going to teach me out there?"

I was so upset that my voice was cracking. I had gone to war for this man, and he was prepared to discard me like an old uniform. I looked at him and saw nothing. No feeling, no concern, no discernible emotion at all. I knew that my days as a Steeler were numbered.

Without telling the Steelers, I went to Jefferson Hospital for another medical opinion. I knew that Chuck and the club officials would have been furious had they known; it's a major no-no for any player to think too much on his own. They prefer the player to be a violent monster on the field, but a docile dog/child/robot (pick one) off it.

The doctor at Jefferson told me about all these new drugs that he could inject into my knee to take away some of the pain, if I so desired.

"Your knee problems," the hospital doctor said, "basically seem to be those of attrition. I can't tell for sure unless I scope around." (Scope: sports medicine vernacular for arthroscopic surgery. It was a revolutionary procedure: in and out of the hospital in hours, in and out of the rehab room in weeks.) He also said that major damage could result if I continued playing.

This, by the way, was not the opinion of the Steeler physician, who had concluded that there was nothing significantly wrong with the knee.

I went to practice the next day and spoke to assistant coach Bill Meyers. I told him that this was the worst injury I'd ever had, and that another doctor had confirmed this for me.

Meyers continued to badmouth me on the sidelines, while Mike Webster tried to defend me.

"Steve is not the type of guy to fake an injury," Webbie said, adding that every injury is different and I was obviously a player who had previously played in pain—perhaps the ultimate compliment for a football player—so why not lay off and "give him a break." But Meyers basically ignored both of us.

At lunchtime I went to the weight room, figuring I could work off some of my frustration. If I couldn't lift with my legs, I'd at least be able to do some upper-body reps. I had barely begun my bench-press routine when Jon Kolb came over.

"Have you talked to Chuck lately?" he said. "I think you may need to see him." Just then Tony Parisi, the equipment manager, stuck his head in and said, "Chuck wants to see you in his office."

Chuck must really be pissed, I thought. One was rarely given an audience with the great man, and I had seen him only a few days before.

I walked into Chuck's office. He was sitting behind his desk, looking as distant and forbidding as ever. He wasted no time with amenities.

"Steve, we just traded you to Tampa Bay for Ray Snell," he said. "Thanks for the seven years."

He shook my hand and showed me the door.

I was numb. I don't even remember walking out of Chuck's office and into the hallway. Dick Haley, director of player personnel, was waiting there for me.

"Phil Krueger is on the phone," Haley said. "He wants to talk to you." Krueger was Tampa's assistant to president (and coach) John McKay. Phil said that the Bucs wanted me down there right away, and that they were glad to get a player of my caliber.

I was still in shock. Barely a month before, I had signed a three-year deal with the Steelers even though the Houston Gamblers of the USFL had offered more money (a similar salary structure, but $65,000 more in up-front money). For a while, I was thinking seriously about gambling on the Gamblers; the thought of being a pioneer had some appeal.

But in the end, primarily out of familiarity and loyalty, I chose to remain with the Steelers.

After I got off the phone with Phil Krueger, I walked down the corridor past the coaches' room. Chuck was in there with all his assistants; they could hear my footsteps on the floor, and they all looked up as I walked back. And just as quickly, they all turned away. Not one of those cleat-licking invertebrates came out to shake my hand. They ignored me like I had the plague. I will never forget that.

Some of these men were my friends. Yet not one of them had the brass to look me in the face and wish me well. Not one of them wanted to buck their head coach. Not one of them was willing to do the right thing.

I went to my room to clear out my gear, and the reporters were swarming around, asking questions. I tried my best to suppress my bitterness. I told them that I had had seven good years with the Steelers, but that I didn't know if I had any more football in my knee.

My buddies on the line and I had frequently talked about what we would do if our parting from the Steelers was, let's say, anything but sweet. We talked about driving our four-wheel-drive vehicles—each of us owned one—across the field, past a scurrying-for-cover Chuck and his weasel assistants, and ramming down one of the goalposts. We'd then rev up on our back wheels like a bucking stallion and ride off in a cloud of dust.

After I cleaned out my stuff and left the reporters, I climbed into my camouflage Blazer and honked the horn. I saw my buddies—Dunn and Webbie—scrambling to get as far away from Chuck as they could.

Instead of any grand parting gesture, however, I just honked again and waved.

There was probably no way to avoid the disappointment and anger I felt toward the Steelers with the way they handled my leave-taking. I put my body and soul on the line for these people. I did everything they asked me to, including jeopardizing my future health. I gave seven years of maximum effort. And all I wanted in return was a simple "thank you."

Maybe that sounds simpy or sappy, but I don't think that some courtesy or loyalty was too much to ask. Coaches and teams are always giving lip service to the concept of loyalty. Yet in Steelerville, with few exceptions, loyalty was a street that ran one way.

I reported to Tampa the next day not knowing if I could play, not knowing if I really wanted to. I was disillusioned with the game. Every player tries to tell himself that football is a business, that it's a cold, cruel world more likely to bruise bones than feelings. But I was definitely hurt—inside and out.

The trade was conditional on me passing a physical. The Tampa doctors examined my knee and did find some moving objects in there—bone and cartilage chips. They said that with arthroscopic surgery I should be okay, and could probably play in about four weeks.

Obviously I felt some vindication. In Pittsburgh, just a few days before, I read in the papers that Chuck felt that my injury might be in my head.

The Tampa physicians' diagnosis was accurate; it took nearly a month to get the knee feeling right. But with rest and rehab, the knee felt better. I was learning a new system. And I was excited about playing football again.

I was also juiced.

For the first time in my career, I cycled anabolic-androgenic steroids *during* the season—basically to facilitate recuperation from knee surgery, so my legs wouldn't atrophy and I could rebuild them more quickly.

I started the third game of the season against the Lions, in which I faced off against Doug English, an All-Pro defensive tackle and a very tough opponent. I couldn't get any real rhythm. I had had only one week of practice in shorts, and one more in pads. For about one fourth of the plays, I had to ask a teammate what to do.

The following week we were to play the Giants—with a tremendous corps of linebackers anchored by the fierce and talented Lawrence Taylor. Playing beside me at left tackle was Gene Sanders, a converted defensive lineman. His technique was still a bit spotty, particularly his hand technique. But he was a big kid—around 290 pounds—with quick feet. I remembered how difficult an adjustment I had when I came into the league, and I thought I could help Gene with a few pointers.

But Kim Helton, our offensive line coach, was not too thrilled with my moonlighting as a de facto coach.

"You're having enough trouble learning the plays, Courson," he basically said. "Stick to your side of the field."

For some reason Helton would often ridicule my performance and belittle me personally. I believed that he resented me because I didn't fit into the mold. At this point, I had developed a reputation as something of a free thinker, and that isn't much appreciated by the would-be military men who are looking for unquestioning foot soldiers. Anything or anyone different is reviled.

I also believe that he was threatened by me because I had played on a world champion, because I had made the Pro Bowl, and because he was afraid that I might usurp his authority with the younger players.

To me, Kim Helton represented the quintessential *assistant* football coach—lacking the real stones to lead, he served as the head man's lackey, badmouthing rather than encouraging, yelling at players rather than trying to teach them. Helton was your typical Southern cracker who favored clichés such as "Go out there and knock a hole through them, men!" Or: "Throw your hats into the ring!"

He was also the kind of guy who demanded that his players refer to him as Coach Helton. C'mon, Kimmie. Even Charles Noll let his players call him Chuck.

The Giants beat us badly that week, and Lawrence Taylor got four sacks. No excuses, but a couple of them were because Gene and I hadn't played much together.

After the game the New York press descended into our locker room and began blowing Lawrence Taylor out of all human proportion, basically just kissing his ass. Don't get me wrong: I think the guy is one of the great linebackers of all time. But that day they said he just ate us alive, and I believe that we just beat ourselves.

Over in the corner, Coach Helton was silently evaluating my performance with some of the nastiest looks I'd ever seen. If he could have gotten away with smacking me around the room, I believe he would have. But I was definitely not in the mood for his psycho-pseudo military bullshit, and I remember thinking, *One word and I dust him.* I also thought, *One overhand right, and my NFL career is dust.* So I turned the other cheek and just walked the other way.

About halfway through the year I got to know the system inside and out, my knee was in great shape, and I was still feeling the stimulating effects of my last cycle. After the game against the 49ers, in which I had played well, I was talking in the locker room to Paul Zimmerman of *Sports Illustrated.* Zimmerman, whose football analysis I always respect, commented to me: "You know, Steve, you should still be in Pittsburgh."

"You're right, Z," I said. Standing right beside us was Kim Helton, who apparently relayed this exchange to his bosses. Sure enough, the following week I was told that Coach McKay was not happy with my progress and that I would no longer be starting.

But after a week or two in the doghouse, I shook off the

fleas and eventually won back my job. The season eventually ended on a high note—with us decisively beating the Falcons and Jets the last two games, both of which I started and kicked butt.

So I began the off-season with a renewed sense of purpose. After eight years in the NFL, though, I knew that I'd have to step up my training regimen if I wanted to compete at the same level. And that included stepping up the chemical dosage.

That off-season, I moved to Boulder, Colorado, and trained six days a week, twice a day. In the mornings, I worked on bench presses, inclines, dead lifts, and squats. In the evenings, I worked on assistance muscles, doing leg extensions, triceps, and weighted dips. I also tried to isolate, and then work on, specific muscles.

Using Fred Hatfield's book, *Bodybuilding: A Scientific Approach*, as a primer, I cycled his recommended dose pattern of anabolic steroids and human chorionic gonadotropin (to stimulate testosterone levels). I also decided to compete in my first weightlifting competition, the Colorado State Powerlifting Championships, in the 275-pound weight class. In order make that weight, I had to lose twenty pounds in two weeks.

I hate diets for two reasons: I like food, and I love beer. But, in addition to the incentive of a new competitive challenge, I was motivated to train for one more reason: I looked forward to exchanging information about AAS cycles with the other lifters. Even if I bombed out, I could probably pick up a few helpful hints.

I finished second in my weight class, raising 745 pounds in the dead lift and barely missing out on the state record of 775 pounds. I was really excited by this sport. It was fun, challenging, and could only help with my football training.

Preparing for the Bucs' April minicamp, I began my most serious cycle yet: a weekly regimen of 4 cc testosterone cypionate, 4cc Winstrol V, 4 cc Deca-Durabolin, and 4 cc liquid Dianabol. I knew that it was a lot, but it seemed worth the risk, and I had yet to experience any major negative side effects. My intention was to enter the '85 season at 285 pounds—able to bench press more than 600 pounds, squat about 850, and dead lift about 900.

The Bucs' preseason physical was routine. The doctors tested hearing, sight, blood, urine, heart, and old joint wounds. Dr. Diaco, the team physician, told me that I'd be taking a blood test to check liver functions—a procedure for those players who may be using anabolic-androgenic steroids. It's an excellent idea, utilized by few teams, which are mostly under the NFL-mandated impression that no player in the league is even thinking about taking steroids.

It was good to be back in the locker room, schmoozing with my teammates. After lunch I was sitting by my locker when Jay Shoop, the Bucs' new trainer, came by to inform me that the morning tests indicated an "abnormality" in my electrocardiogram. There was nothing to be concerned about, he said; but just to be sure, I'd be seeing a cardiologist in Tampa. Immediately.

As soon as I got there, they hooked me up to an electrocardiogram machine; this time I was laid flat on a table while the nurse monitored the printout. I couldn't see the monitor or her pad, but I could read the note of concern on her face.

During the consultation, the cardiologist asked me if I drank or took any medication. There was no purpose in lying. "Yes," I told him. "I drink a lot of beer. And right now I'm in the middle of a substantial AAS cycle." I told him the drugs and the dosage.

"You've got to stop taking these drugs immediately," he said. My resting heart rate, he informed me, was 160 beats per minute. (The norm is about 70–72.)

On the car ride back to team headquarters at 1 Buccaneer

Place, I was confused and scared; my mind was racing. I wondered if all the drugs I had taken in order to compete were destroying my body. I always wondered if there would be any consequences. I had thought that I was young and strong and impervious to something as mundane as mortality—football or otherwise.

I decided at that moment to retire. I immediately went in to see the Bucs' new head coach, Leeman Bennett.

"I'm just playing for the money, Coach," I told him. "It's not fair to my teammates, to you, and to myself." I also told him that my frustration was causing me to drink more heavily than usual. What I didn't say to Leeman Bennett or G.M. Phil Krueger, whom I spoke to next, was that the game didn't seem worth the effort anymore; that, in the lust for winning and success, I had lost perspective. I didn't say it, but they'd be fools not to think it: This little scare had been a major shock, and not only to my cardiological system.

I guess you could say my heart just wasn't in it.

At this point the doctors were telling me that my condition would soon revert back to normal. With proper medication, I could be back to training again. And though the doctors did not specifically blame the atrial fibrillation (the clinical term for the abnormality) on my steroid usage, it was my belief that the recent excessive cycle had probably precipitated it. For the first time, I reflected on my situation and reevaluated the risks of continued steroid usage.

Then I observed an incident that would prove even more disturbing. While unloading my gear from the local health club locker room, I stumbled into two young football players giving each other injections of testosterone. These kids couldn't have been more than 16 years old. I was too dumbfounded to say anything to them. I sort of mumbled something and slunk out.

Until that moment, I never realized how widespread the use of steroids had become. I didn't even think that kids that age could be involved. As an adult, I had found ways to rationalize the use of these chemicals in order to make a living: I had a job to do, and steroids helped me do it. There was no way, however, that I could justify a 16-year-old using these same drugs.

I wondered if I was in some way responsible. Wasn't I supposed to be a role model? Didn't youngsters take their cues from professional athletes? If we were so blasé about taking these drugs—and let's face it, contrary to NFL pronouncements, kids do know that we're taking them—how could we expect them to do as we say, not as we do?

So when a writer for *Sports Illustrated* contacted me for a special report on anabolic-androgenic steroid use in the NFL, I couldn't just say no. And when asked if I was currently using steroids, I simply said, "Yes, I am."

If I knew then what effect that honest response would have on the rest of my life, would I give the same answer again?

Probably. But back then nothing could have prepared me for the minifirestorm of controversy that engulfed the professional football world, and my little place in it.

7

THE
ARTICLE
AND ITS
AFTERMATH

WHEN IN THE spring of 1985 Jill Lieber, a writer at *Sports Illustrated*, called and asked me to talk at length about my steroid usage, I was at a particularly vulnerable time in my life. I had recently—and perhaps rashly—chosen to give up the sport that had been the focal point of my life for the past 18 years. I hadn't yet decided what I was going to do next. The Bucs had just contacted my agent and wanted me to return to the team. And while I was thinking about playing again, I got the call that changed my life.

I decided that I would come clean. I would tell as much as I could about my own steroid usage over the years. I would not talk specifically about anyone else's use, and I would not name names. Lieber did say that she was talking to another big-name player who had admitted his current steroid usage, but that he did not want to be quoted in the article by name.

"Would you speak on the record?" she asked.

"Yes," I said.

We talked for twelve hours over several days. It was kind of a kick for me. I, of course, had been interviewed many times before by the local media, but had never been the primary focus of a major article in a national magazine. For an offensive lineman, it was a hell of an ego massage. It was also fun to strut around topless for a photographer, who said he wanted to get the full effect of my AAS-enhanced physique.

The conversations were a lot like therapy and, like most confessions, seemed good for my soul. I was asked if, of all team sports, drugs in football were the worst. Although I had no firsthand experience in other professional sports, I said this was probably true. The more pain and injury there is in a sport, the more likely that drugs are going to be used.

The article, a first-person narrative distilled from our conversations, was the second of three parts in a *Sports Illustrated* special report called "Steroids: A Problem of Huge Dimensions."

The third part was on Charles J. Radler, at one time the biggest dealer of anabolic steroids in the country (grossing $20,000 a week), who was then serving time in jail. The first part was sort of an overview on steroid use in pro football, with *S.I.* correspondents interviewing 25 then-active NFL players—only two of whom admitted to currently using steroids. One was the anonymous player Lieber had mentioned; the other was, of course, me.

Statements on the issue ranged widely, depending on who was being quoted—and who and what they had to protect. Fred Smerlas, a Buffalo Bills nose tackle, said that he thought 40 percent of NFL players were using steroids. Gene Upshaw, a former offensive lineman with the Raiders and now the executive director of the NFL Players Association, said for the record: "I never knew any guys who took steroids. . . . There's no black market of steroids. . . . I don't think steroids are a problem in the NFL." And one week before the report was published in *S.I.*, NFL commissioner Pete Rozelle was quoted: "I feel confident that steroids are not being dispensed to any heavy degree by the clubs. But you can't stop someone from getting them on the outside. We tell them, first, it's debatable as to whether or not it improves performance and, second, we tell them about potential side effects. I don't think steroid use is that big—with the clubs not dispensing steroids and with athletes not being overly prone to buy it if they have to pay for it."

Then, of course, a page or two later, Ol' Can't Keep His Trap Shut Courson gave his own facts, figures, notes, and quotes: "Seventy-five percent of the linemen in the NFL are on steroids and 95 percent have probably tried them. Even in college, they're widely used. Rookies, at every training camp, have asked me about them. Most of them have tried some kind of steroid."

Then I said: "What's wrong with a football player building his body as strong as he can with steroids? I know I have to play a 16-game season, and to survive without serious injury I have to be as strong as I can possibly be."

And similarly: "Football is my business. I take this attitude towards drugs: They give me an edge in my business. I don't regret anything I've done so far as pharmaceutical use is concerned. It's very easy for people on the outside to criticize. But it's different when it's your livelihood, when it's your job to keep a genetic mutation from getting into your backfield."

I also said: "In order to compete at this business, you absolutely have to know the pluses and minues that come along with using steroids. Maybe kidney and liver disease when you're older."

And, in what was to become an even more chilling statement in light of my subsequent medical history, I said: "But you do what you have to do, otherwise you don't have your job. I don't want to leave this game broken and crippled. And, I know that, with steroids, I have less chance of being broken and crippled because I was stronger."

All my comments, thankfully, were not as flip: "Of course, anyone who uses steroids wants more research done. We want to know what we'll be facing 50, 60—even 20—years from now. Then it will be easier to make a concrete choice about using steroids. Right now, there's an X factor. You don't know what the X factor is, but you do know you're reaping benefits."

Until that time, no active or former NFL player had spoken as loudly or at such length (or by name) about his steroid usage. Most athletes have difficulty accepting that they may have needed an artificial boost to compete. They also feel that such an admission would minimize their achievements. Many athletes, unfortunately, have their self-esteem tied into performance: they play well, they feel good; they play badly, they feel lousy.

I know many pro football players—and several I played with—who point their fingers in self-righteous indignation at steroid users, while conveniently forgetting their own use of amphetamines or painkillers; somehow, in their minds, those drugs don't constitute "cheating."

Few athletes want to acknowledge, even to themselves, that drugs may have had an influence—no matter how marginal—on their success. And yet that tiny margin can be the difference between a silver or a gold, or no medal at all. Just think how one second, one inch, or even one missed tackle can affect someone's life.

How many of us can resist such enormous temptation?

What was unique about my so-called confession was that I had not been caught "cheating." I was not one of those guys who'd been popped for drugs and had nothing to lose by baring his soul except a few months off his prison sentence. Nor did I do it for the money; *Sports Illustrated* did not pay a penny for my thoughts or my time. Why then did I choose to come forward and speak openly about these things?

No doubt seeing those two high school kids shooting up was a factor. But I had my own reasons. With the recent heart scare, I was concerned about my health, about the X factor, and I thought if someone addressed these issues, that could be the first step toward increased knowledge about the risks. I was also tired of the sporting establishment's laissez-faire attitude that only seemed to perpetuate an almost universal conspiracy of silence.

I took these drugs voluntarily and unashamedly, but I also felt compelled by the system. Most of my competition was using these drugs; how could I afford not to?

Taking steroids was a big part of my work and my life, and an integral part of the game. I could not deny that any longer, to myself or to anyone else.

All these reasons were factored into my decision to talk, but at the time I didn't really consider all the ramifications. I did begin to think then, though, that there might be a little problem with the Bucs if I did choose to return to football. So when Jill Lieber called me a few days later to confirm my quotes, I specifically told her to be careful in choosing the material to include; it could cost me my career. I did not, however, disavow any of the comments, nor tell her what to, or what not to, write.

After some further discussions with the Bucs, I decided to attend the team's second minicamp. Boarding the plane to Tampa at Stapleton Airport in Denver, I picked up the May 13, 1985, issue of *Sports Illustrated*. In the center of the magazine, complete with beefcake photos of my bare-chested torso, was the gist of my conversations with Jill Lieber. There was nothing in there that I hadn't said, though it read a little colder and more inflammatory than I had intended.

The reaction, though greater than I had anticipated, was predictable. The Bucs' organization was definitely not pleased with my sudden notoriety. Perhaps as a result of receiving pressure from "upstairs," Tampa Bay trainer Jay Shoop told me to consider a retraction.

Of what, I wondered. "Sorry, folks, I didn't really mean to say those things. I really meant to lie."

My teammates and other NFL players basically applauded me for telling the truth, though several commented that I may have had "more balls than brains."

It was pretty lonely out there, as I soon became a target of every crackpot on both sides of the issue. The fans and media either praised me for my candor, or often viciously denounced me for my "drug abuse."

Sports Illustrated may have raised its circulation, as well as a few questions, with all the controversy. But nothing much changed—certainly not the league policy on steroids.

Instead, the poobahs and spinmeisters at Pete Rozelle's NFL, Inc., opted for damage control, issuing a brief flurry of innocuous P.R. releases before resuming business as usual.

"If a player is attempting to enhance his performance on the field by anabolic steroids, it's wrong," said Rozelle immediately following the article. Mr. Rozelle also sicced one of his minions on me, purportedly to gauge my reasons for speaking out about steroids, but more likely to set my mind "right."

The meeting itself, with Warren Walsh of the NFL's Security Commission, was pleasant enough. I had met Walsh before, when he and his sidekick, Charlie Jackson, had visited our training camps and given us the league's anti-gambling, anti-drug scare speech. They used to tell us how they were there to protect us against the many sinister elements in society that would try to exploit us.

This time, Warren and I discussed the positive and negative aspects of steroid uses. Then he asked me: "Steve, have you ever thought that it wasn't fair to take steroids?"

Fair?!? I "fairly" exploded at the implications of that question.

Is it fair that players are expected to take painkilling needles on the advice of a single team physician? Is it fair that NFL offensive lineman are treated like second-class citizens in terms of recognition and financial compensation? Is it fair that number-one draft picks are paid more in signing bonuses than some established players make in a career? Is it fair that a crippling injury would end that career tomorrow, without so much as a fare-thee-well?

What right does the NFL have to bring up the issue of fairness?

In all *fairness*, it wasn't Warren Walsh's fault that he had no clue to comprehending a player's mindset. He was just another suit doing his job. One couldn't expect men who make their living in ties and white shirts to know what it's like out there in helmet and pads. But his lack of understanding mirrored the thinking of the NFL and, unfortunately, some of the public as well.

After the publication of the *S.I.* article, the Bucs made their own attempts to get my mind right. Once a week, they sent me to Dr. Klein, a psychologist. Maybe they thought I was crazy for telling the truth.

Dr. Klein seemed a competent enough therapist and a decent fellow, but he too hadn't a clue when it came to anabolic steroids. Had his questions gone deeper than the typical layperson's (Are you still taking steroids? Why did you take them? Do you have the desire to take them again? Couldn't you have gotten the same results without them?), then perhaps I might have learned a few things about my psychological dependence on these drugs. As it was, I passed a few pleasant 45-minute hours without gaining much, if any, insight.

I found it pretty amusing that because of my admitted steroid use, I was now being sent to a psychologist. What about all that time when I had consumed significant amounts of steroids (with the team's knowledge) without saying a word? What about all those years when I blindly accepted painkilling needles and drugs? And what about every one of those days in football games or practices when I flung my body into huge, angry, charging men who could, at any moment, break any number of my bones? If any behavior warranted a visit to a shrink, it was any one of the above.

I suppose I could have looked at these mandatory sessions as either management's sincere attempt to provide help or as a subtle form of brainwashing.

Around this time, I received an offer to participate in the Jack Lambert Football Camp. It was the first chance I had had in more than six months to return to the Pittsburgh area. It was great to see some of my old teammates, particularly the always-ready-to-party Gary Dunn, as well as to get in some hands-on coaching experience with the kids. (It also gave me an opportunity to stop in at my tailor in Pittsburgh and order some new threads. With my bizarre measurements—waist, 38½"; chest, 58"; biceps, 20½"; thighs, 29"; neck, 22¾"—finding clothes was always a problem. I'd often rip the sleeves of my shirts and jackets just by putting them on. There wasn't too many off-the-rack items that could suit this sort of frame.)

There was and is something about Pittsburgh that's special to me. Maybe it was having spent the better part of my rowdy youth there. Maybe it was being part of the most successful team in the city's sports history. Maybe it was just relating to the rock-solid values and down-to-earth attitude of the people. I didn't realize how much I missed the city until I returned for a visit. I knew then that I'd probably come back to live there someday.

When I returned to Tampa for what would be my final season in the NFL, I thought a lot about my steroid use. Obviously I don't know for sure if I could have achieved the same success in the NFL without the use of steroids. But I do believe I could have excelled—though probably, with my speed and natural weight, at linebacker.

I was ready to prove to myself and others that I did not need AAS in order to compete. So I vowed to play clean and trained as hard as I always did. (Even when I was off cycle, I tried to maintain the same rigorous intensity. I just could not recuperate as fast, so my strength wasn't as great.)

The loss of strength and bulk was definitely measurable. On the juice, I could bench press 500 pounds at least six repetitions. Before going into training camp, I was probably benching less than 450 for no more than five reps. Obviously the drop-off would be even greater at the end of the season; after the weekly poundings, some decrease was expected. My weight went down from 295 in my juiced-up prime to about 270 pounds.

The main advantage to being lighter, especially playing in the Florida heat, was that I did not tire as easily. Though the Bucs finished a dismal 2–14, I had a good individual season, as good as I'd ever had. However, I did feel that had I cycled steroids, I probably could have played even better.

After the season, neither the front office nor the coaches gave me any indication whether they wanted me back or not. I had one year and an option year left on my contract. I, too, was undecided about playing in Tampa. It wasn't much fun participating in a losing program after seven years with the Steelers. Nor did I much care for the coaching methods at Tampa Bay, mainly due to my still-icy relations with line coach Kim Helton.

Even though I was finding it so much harder to get pumped—physically and mentally—for the game, I was sufficiently motivated to train clean and hard for about three or four months in the off-season.

Maybe it because I was finally feeling my football mortality. Maybe it was just trying to get it up for one final campaign. Maybe it was because I felt so beaten up psychologically and physiologically. Mostly it was because I had learned the irrefutable lesson that drugs definitely helped you recuperate faster.

For whatever the reason—and I'm still not proud of it—I decided to go on a light AAS cycle. Nothing too androgenic, I figured, since I wanted to avoid muscle pulls, so I took a mild dose of Winstrol V and Deca-Durabolin. I was definitely worried about getting hurt, and I thought that by not being as explosive and powerful as I once was, I was more likely to get injured. At least, that was my rationale.

I saw what playing clean and being a crusader meant: squat, nada, zilch. Nobody gave a rat's ass whether I got injured or not. They'd move someone else right in there in a New York minute.

Immediately I felt the difference. By the time I came into minicamp, I was 288 pounds—rock hard and ready to roll. I blew everyone out in the strength tests, and ran really well. Even my old nemesis, Kim Helton, noticed the change— you'd have to be blind not to see that I was a different-looking human than I was the year before, and you'd have to be pretty dumb not to figure out that it was chemically induced. Sean Farrell, the starting left guard, was not in camp, so I got to work out with the varsity.

But after minicamp, I thought to myself: Farrell returns, and I'm back on the bench. Do I want to go through the same crap as last year—the same tired old coaches' tirades, the same tired old dehumanizing meat grinder?

The year before, when I played clean, I vowed not to let

them stick me with any needles; I was not going to take any painkillers to play. I still felt that way, even more so. Which only meant one thing: I was not prepared to pay the price that I had so willingly coughed up for nearly 20 years.

There was one thing that I knew for sure: I wanted out of Tampa Bay. So my agent called the Bucs and requested a trade; he might even have threatened them: Trade Steve or he files a grievance with the union (though I'm not sure on what grounds).

Two weeks later, the Bucs released me. The reasons they gave were that I had been beaten out by a younger player, and I had been unproductive the previous year. If anyone had checked the stats, however, they would have seen that I had given up the fewest sacks on the team.

I had been a Pro Bowl alternate for the Steelers in '82, and I would say my final year in Tampa Bay was equivalent. I knew I could still play. And, as soon as they said I couldn't play, I knew that I wanted to. I assumed that someone would give me the opportunity.

Only two people called after Tampa Bay waived me: my dad and Mike Webster. My father was real angry at the way the Bucs treated me. Webbie had been around a while; he had seen many of his teammates and friends come and go. He was more philosophical, though still very supportive. He knew I could still play if I wanted to.

Not one NFL team called. Not one offer to come to training camp. Not even a tryout. I looked around at some of the retreads they were bringing in to camp for a look-see. After nine productive years in pro football, there was not one team in the league that could take a no-risk chance on my services? A more paranoid sort—though some have certainly labeled me as such—would have thought there was some unofficial blackballing going on.

Maybe they felt that I was still a little too hot to handle. I was known as that "steroid guy," a whistle-blower and, even worse, a free thinker. Certainly the NFL has never been known for being in the vanguard of enlightened thought.

I went to Myrtle Beach for a month, hoping someone still might call. I worked out with weights and ran every day. I also sat around on the beach a lot, sadly contemplating my future. I was one sorry sack of beef.

I was even sorrier when I returned home and my agent told me that no one had called. It was getting on into late summer, and the season was gearing up. It was the first time in eighteen years that I would not be putting on pads.

In September, the Bucs issued a short statement announcing my official retirement from football. Soon after, for the first fall vacation of my life, I flew to Munich for Oktoberfest.

When I returned from Germany, I remember sitting in the cab thinking, What the hell am I going to do with the rest of my life? I was barely 30, and it seemed like I had nowhere to go, nothing I really wanted to do.

I rented a cabin in Wyoming and began taking notes for a possible book, as much for therapy as for publication. Ironically, it was Jill Lieber who first suggested that I think about writing a book someday. No doubt she thought of it primarily in terms of the steroid issue, and indeed that's how it began, with me doing an enormous amount of research on the subject.

While in Wyoming considering my past, there was one more big dose of irony: Right before the '87 Orange Bowl, Brian Bosworth of Oklahoma tested positive for steroids, and the media fell over themselves trying to get in touch with me. They knew I was one of the few professional athletes, present or past, who would talk openly and honestly about the issue. I became several journalists' pet expert on the topic, giving juicy quotes as well as solid background. I knew my stuff.

When the furor over the Boz died down, so did the media's interest in me. I had no job, no real direction, and virtually no clue. I couldn't stop wallowing in frustration and self-pity.

I felt that nothing had gone right for me since the *S.I.* article. I had broken the cardinal rule of professional athletes: Don't get caught, and don't tell the truth. I was doubly stupid: I came clean without having gotten caught.

I was also very bitter. There's probably no avoiding some bitterness, or bittersweetness, once the glory days are done, for any player. You're young, invincible, playing at the height of your athletic powers. Then, at some point, your skills erode and your short shelf line as an athlete begins to expire. You can't avoid wishing it were otherwise—that those intense intoxicating Sundays could continue for more than just a handful of years. Like the song says: You don't know what you've got till it's gone.

Let me tell you: It goes too damn soon.

Many athletes are not trained to do much of anything else, and it's a real shock when that realization hits—in essence, when their real life begins. It's not easy to find a replacement for that missing level of excitement, or to become as motivated about pursuing more mundane career opportunities.

How do you fill a void as big as an empty stadium?

I was certainly not alone. Many of my friends and former teammates have had some difficulty adapting to civilian life. Let's face it: for three, six, nine years, we were in our own world. Millions of people watched as we made our bodies into weapons and then went out and hammered our colleagues. We were paid to get as big and strong and fast as we could, and then to hit people as hard as we could.

The adjustments were physical as well as psychological.

I recall a player's association dinner at which 70 percent of the ex-players limped up to receive their awards.

There seems to be a lack of real counseling for NFL players. Both management and the players' association are to blame; neither group has made sufficient efforts to deal with the problem.

One of the reasons I've been so open about my health problems is to jar the NFL into taking action to protect its veterans. When we're young, we put our bodies on the line for our teams. The least they can do is help us maintain them when we're older.

In my case, I lost a half million dollars in bad investments because of an unscrupulous agent; I couldn't even afford the most basic health care premiums. Is it unreasonable to expect the NFL to provide lifetime catastrophe health care for any player with a minimum term of service?

I was overwhelmed with the loss of my livelihood, my income, my athletic youth. The only time I felt in some control, believe it or not, was when I had an alcoholic buzz on. And I was plenty buzzed. Almost every night I was out partying with friends, though the drinking during this period was not like it was during the heart of my career—it was rarely celebratory.

One of my drinking buddies was also a steroid user, and on Halloween, in a 'roid-and-beer attack, he punched out a lawyer, of all people. As part of his rehabilitation, he began going to Alcoholics Anonymous. I saw how it helped him. And then one day he said to me: "I think you have a drinking problem too, partner."

So I went to A.A. I didn't like it. It was humiliating and difficult, particularly for one who was never that interested in self-analysis. My attitude was: Gladiators don't whine (and they definitely don't *schmooze*). But the program was good for me; it made me take a clear-eyed look at my life and how I was letting it get away from me.

I did not believe, however, that I was an alcoholic.

I didn't really match up with the typical alcoholic profile. I had rarely been late for work, never started a fight in a bar, did not drink every day. In fact, during the program I went ninety days without a drink, and it wasn't a big deal; I barely missed it. So I began thinking that maybe I did have a drinking problem and needed to stop drinking, but that alcoholism really wasn't my primary problem.

As a player, I used to drink to excess. Many of my Steeler teammates did as well. Our attitude was: Fight hard all day, drink hard all night. We were proud of that. It was all part of being a tough guy, a macho stud in the testoterone-rich world of pro football. I was a big guy and I could consume considerable quantities without getting roaring, sloppy drunk. Not too many of my teammates could consume as much—only Gary Dunn could keep up—though it didn't stop a good number of them from trying.

In my naïveté (or learned stupidity), I thought this was a big part of being a man. Drinking someone under the table was the stuff of warrior legend. And back then I thought I was immortal. I was beginning to learn that it could all end tomorrow.

Which, of course, it almost did.

8

HEARTS
AND FLOWERS

BY THE SPRING of 1988, I was flat broke. My agent, Greg Lustig, had involved me—and perhaps twenty other Steelers—in a series of limited partnerships, 80 percent of which went belly up; the other 20 percent were unsuitable for my needs. I lost more than $500,000. After enduring all the crap in pro football—nine years of blood, sweat, and more blood—I had nothing to show for it except a few trophies and a couple of Super Bowl rings.

I sold off everything except the trophies and rings and moved back to Pittsburgh. Soon after, in the summer of '88, the Internal Revenue Service came after me for its chunk.

I was probably the second sorriest soul on the planet. The first had to be Ben Johnson. And, as everyone now knows, it was steroids that precipitated his fall.

Right after winning the 100-meter race in Seoul—blowing past Carl Lewis and everyone else to earn the coveted title of "World's Fastest Human"—Johnson tested positive for stanozolol (or its brand name, Winstrol V). His reputation, career, and earning potential were in shambles. It was estimated that he cost himself upwards of $18 million in endorsement income. Other than a few Bulgarian weightlifters, who, uncharacteristically, were also caught, few knew as well as I did just how bad Ben must have felt. I would have had considerably more respect for him, however, had he admitted his mistake and not kept trying to deny it to the public—and perhaps to himself as well.

Johnson's financial losses were enormous, but they were of *potential* earnings. My debts were out of pocket and could not be readily recouped. Other than football, I didn't know of too many legitimate professions in which one could make that kind of dough. And without a college degree and with few marketable skills, it would be difficult for me to earn even a moderately decent wage.

The best way, I thought, to refeather my nest was to pursue a career in the wrestling ring. I figured I could make a lot of money fast and then get out. I had no intentions of being a buffoon for long.

I began learning the ropes from an old-time wrestler, Dominick Denucci, who walked me through some of the basic holds and moves. In a short time, I was ready for my first match, in Charleroi, a small town about 20 miles south of Pittsburgh. Also on the card that night were Tony Atlas and the Sheik, a couple of big names in the "sport." My bout that night was against the Blue Cyclone.

After only three days of practice, they didn't want to give me anything too complicated. So the Cyclone and I basically followed the script to the letter: I gave him a couple of hip tosses, threw him off the ropes, lifted him, body-slammed him to the canvas, and then covered him up. Bing-bang-boom. In no time I had squashed his butt for my first wrestling "victory."

I was the good guy.

At around the same time, I also began training for a

weightlifting meet—a regional tournament in Pittsburgh that was to be held on September 10, 1988, nearly two years to the day since my retirement from football.

Years before, people had tried to discourage me from competitive lifting. They said that my arms were too long. Longer arms mean a longer way to push the weight, and most of the great lifters have short, stubby arms for better leverage. But that only gave me more incentive. There weren't many people in the world who'd bench pressed more than 600 pounds, and that was my goal.

Although it was contrary to everything that I believed in, I continued to take steroids. I wanted to compete at the same level as everyone else, and I knew there was only one way to do that.

By the day of the contest, I was at the end of a sixteen-week cycle, having ingested or injected substantial doses of Dianabol, Anavar (both orals), Deca-Durabolin, testoserone enanthate, and testosterone propionate (oil-based injectables) before capping it off with some human chorionic gonadotropin.

My joint soreness disappeared, and my body weight increased 29 pounds, to 309. My body fat was less than 10 percent. For the first time in months, I felt good physically and mentally. I was truly stoked by the possibilities.

Competing in the bench press, I nailed 575 pounds without even breaking a sweat. Then they moved the weight up to 605, and I smoked that on my second attempt. It was a great feeling to have accomplished my goal; it had been a while since I'd felt such exhilaration. Everybody else in my class—superheavyweight—soon dropped out, and I had my first weightlifting victory.

I felt that this was just the beginning. I had done 605 in only my fifth competition (two NFL Strongman contests, a local bench press meet, and the '85 Colorado State Powerlifting Championships, in which I had placed second), and I hadn't even trained properly. With my knowledge of the science, I knew that I had the potential to bulk up to 345 pounds, overcome my long-arms deficiency, and set the world bench press record, which was then 705 pounds.

But the day after the meet, a feeling of hollow victory set in, and then depression. I wasn't too proud of myself for once again rationalizing my steroid use in order to attain success. And since there didn't seem to be any real money in lifting, I knew I'd have to return to wrestling to pay the rent.

I didn't really feel suited for wrestling, temperamentally or physically. I'd never been a natural performer; I'm basically shy. And though many wrestlers very evidently used steroids to yoke up, strength didn't seem to be a real asset. A facility for tumbling and acrobatics was more essential. Despite the ridicule of many sports fans, wrestling does require considerable know-how, flexibility, and agility. I learned to respect many of these performers as athletes, though I also felt the activity itself was silly. It was mock combat (as opposed, of course, to the more *real* warlike aspects of football).

On October 1st, my 33 birthday, I ran into a bunch of friends downtown, and they began buying me shots of alcohol. I knew that I probably shouldn't be drinking. But I couldn't refuse—it was my birthday, after all—and I grabbed this huge picture of tequila-something and chugged the whole thing. Almost immediately I got this queasy feeling. I walked outside the bar and threw up. I hadn't vomited from alcohol since I was in my early twenties. I assumed it was something I had eaten, and didn't give it another thought.

I began training again with Dominick to get ready for some more wrestling matches. Basically I felt fine, though I would become winded easily. I thought I was just out of shape and simply needed to do more cardiovascular exercises. Or maybe I was getting too big and probably should lose a few pounds.

It soon got to the point where I'd be tired just walking up a flight of stairs. Then, in early November, my stomach mysteriously started bloating. It couldn't have been the steroids, since I'd been clean for almost two months. And other than that binge on my birthday, I hadn't done much drinking.

I thought that maybe I had a virus or a mild stomach disorder that would likely pass in time. I also resisted going to a doctor because I really couldn't afford the visit.

I continued to get sicker by the day. The bloating continued. I couldn't keep any food down. Nor could I sleep— mainly because I couldn't stop hiccuping.

Finally, on the day before Thanksgiving, I roused myself out of bed and drove the six miles to Central Medical Hospital, where my rested heart rate was assessed at 200 beats per minute. My blood pressure was 80 over 50. The admitting physician said that I looked gray, deathly.

After my chest x-ray was analyzed, I was taken from the emergency room to intensive care. There, listed in critical condition, I spent Thanksgiving and another three days. The next four I spent traveling in and out of various testing rooms. Subsequently I was told by several doctors and nurses that they never thought I'd last through the first night, much less the week.

I had absolutely no energy, yet I still couldn't sleep. The doctors refused to give me any sleeping pills, because they wanted me to remain coherent; my pain would help them to figure out what was ailing me.

My second night in intensive care, I got a call from a medical reporter at a local Pittsburgh station who wanted to interview me. I wondered how the word had gotten out. It wasn't like the media had been avidly tracking my post-football career. I guess once a Steeler. . . .

I told the doctors to deflect any and all reporters' queries. I did not yet feel that my medical condition was everyone's business.

Dr. Rosenbloom, a cardiologist, took over my case. I was as straight with him as he was with me. I told him about my medical history and genealogy (as much as I knew), my professional history of injuries, and my lengthy history of drug and alcohol use. He told me that the interminable hiccups, which by then had lasted weeks, were likely connected to heart disease—in my case, dilated cardiomyopathy.

"An enlarged heart in which muscle fibers are lost over time," he explained. "Your heart is flabby and baggy and doesn't pump as a normal heart should."

Imagine that: a bulked-up powerlifter with a flabby heart.

He then told me that there were several options, the final—and most likely—being a heart transplant. He also said in typical doctorese that if I maintained my life-style I would soon die.

What he did not immediately tell me was that my life expectancy didn't look all that rosy under the best of circumstances. With a transplant—assuming a heart could be found to accommodate my size—I could expect, on average, an additional five years. Without one, there was— and is—an 80 percent chance that I would die within three to five years.

As of this writing, it is just about three years since Dr. Rosenbloom's diagnosis (and he has yet to send me his bill). In football terms, we're in the middle of the second half, with the clock ticking furiously away.

Prior to that discussion with Dr. Rosenbloom, I'd been thinking that I was a pretty sick boy, but the tough stuff was probably behind me. Hearing the cold, grim prognosis was, needless to say, a shock to my emotional system.

For the previous three months, I had thrown up several

times a day; my weight had gone from 300 to 225 pounds, my lowest weight since I was 17.

Could it get any worse?

To assess whether I was a viable candidate for a heart transplant, I was to be given a rigorous three-day evaluation at Allegheny General Hospital—a test of my psychological as well as physiological suitability. With a week to spare before the evaluation, I went home to Gettysburg to spend some time with my parents. Mom's home cooking, Dad's no-nonsense optimism, and I was soon feeling better.

One morning, the phone rang. "Hi, this is Ed Bouchette of the *Pittsburgh Post-Gazette*.

"Steve, I've been hearing some crazy rumors about your health," he continued. "Something about you needing a heart transplant."

Apparently he had gotten wind of the efforts of some former teammates—primarily Tunch Ilkin and Mike Webster—to raise some money for my medical bills. They were planning a roast in Webbie's name.

(Originally my friends hadn't even told me about the roast; they just went about making plans. All those years we had talked about the special camaraderie born out of the violence and stress of professional football, convincing each other that there were few people you could really count on—most of whom were to be found knee deep and side by side in the same "trench." My buddies were certainly there when I needed them. Around this same time, Tunch Ilkin informed Dan Rooney of the Steelers about my health problems. Dan expressed his regrets, and the Steelers assured the fundraising committee that they would buy a table at the upcoming roast. To this day, for whatever reasons, the Steelers have not yet paid for their table.)

I've always been a straight shooter with reporters; they asked me a question, I gave them an honest answer. I never had the energy or the inclination to play politician or diplomat. So when Bouchette asked me if I thought that steroids had played a role in my illness, I said: "Of course it's possible . . ." And then I added, "But we just don't know yet. The research is not there." But I knew that those last few words were lost in the ozone. The savvy reporter already had his story: EX-STEELER FACES DEATH, STEROID ABUSE THE CAUSE.

I spoke to Mike Webster immediately after the interview and told him that I had finally revealed my situation to the media. "Steve," Webbie said, "you know they're going to hang you for this. They're gonna make it look like you did this to yourself."

I already knew that. I remembered the distortions and quarter-truths generated from the *Sports Illustrated* story. I understood that the press didn't really care about *me*. It was a juicy story that had all the elements: drugs, sports, and, for some additional drama, the threat of death.

(On a much bigger—and perhaps more tragic—scale, Lyle Alzado went through a very similar onslaught after his T-cell lymphoma was diagnosed and he soon went public— baring his soul in a first-person article in *Sports Illustrated* and on half a dozen talk shows. One key difference was that Lyle blamed steroids outright for his brain cancer, while I only say that they were "contributing factors" to my cardiomyopathy.)

At Webbie's insistence, I asked anyone wanting to do a story on me to call Dr. Rosenbloom. "I'll authorize him to tell you anything you want to know," I said. "All I ask is that you listen to what he has to say and try not to simplify or sensationalize."

Some simplified, some sensationalized. Several reporters called my doctor, but many decided they had sufficient medical training to make their own determinations. One local media personality, Bruce Keiden, aired his views on me during a radio sports talk show. From what I was told, he felt that my admitted steroid use should lower my status on the transplant list. Perhaps, he suggested, I might not even be worthy of consideration. "Courson did this to himself," Keiden supposedly maintained. "He knew the risks."

Soon after that, a headline in the *Atlanta Constitution* read: AVID ABUSER NOW IN LINE FOR A NEW HEART. The piece also ascribed responsibility on my part for the cardiomyopathy.

After interviewing me on TV, a local sportscaster, Sam Nover, suggested that I would never have made it in the NFL without performance-enhancing drugs. Sam, of course, was basing his expert opinion on decades of medical training, not to mention a lifetime of experience as a professional football scout, coach, and player. Just think: You, too, can be transformed from ignorant yahoo to Renaissance man in a few short months with only a microphone and some vocal chords.

I wondered: Was it stupidity or venality?

I'm not sure why some people are so quick to castigate pro athletes, and often so cruelly. I suppose we make big, soft targets who (usually) don't hit back. Rarely, too, is an athlete powerful enough to affect the livelihood of a member of the press, but often the league or team management *is* in a position to hire or fire. Might that influence someone's—anyone's—reporting?

It still amazes me that the self-appointed Defenders of Public Decency in and out of the media expect working athletes to know more than the top scientists and physicians, who've admitted that they haven't yet explored the long-term effects of these drugs.

In my case, they only had to ask my doctor.

"I'm more suspicious of a virus," said Dr. Rosenbloom, responding to a writer from *Sports Illustrated*, noting that AAS use usually results in "a thickening, hypertrophying of the heart"—the opposite of my case. "But we don't know that Steve's condition is not the result of many years of heavy anabolic steroid use," he continued. "We just don't know. There's not that much research."

Overall, most of the fans and the media were fair and supportive in their dealings with me, although, to this day, reporters still ask, "Do you regret your steroid use?"

Sure I do, but not for the reasons they assume.

It's as if they want me to be a poster boy for steroid abuse and flagellate myself in public. They expect me to frighten away potential users with heartrending accounts of my "tragedy."

I refuse to play that game.

Because we just don't *know*, many well-meaning folks have overblown the health effects of steroids, often using gloom-and-doom claims and statistics as a scare tactic. In some cases the claims are wildly irresponsible, not to mention untrue. You cannot persuade people to do the right thing for the wrong reasons.

Take the Biden committee, for example.

In the spring of 1989, Senator Joseph Biden of Delaware convened the Senate Judiciary Committee to debate the proposed Steroid Trafficking Act—a bill that would add steroids to the list of Schedule II controlled substances and "boost the penalties for steroid trafficking, impose tight production controls on pharmaceutical companies and incorporate steroid prevention and treatment programs in our national drug abuse strategy." It was a good bill, yet many of the politicians used it as a forum to advance their own careers, and not the facts.

Many of those who testified as expert witnesses also tried to project—as well as protect—their own agendas. In two full days of hearings, many of the usual suspects were heard from, including Pete Rozelle, Chuck Noll, NFL Players Association President Gene Upshaw, Kansas City Chiefs coach Marty Shottenheimer, and Atlanta Falcons offensive guard Bill Fralic; Olympians such as Evelyn Ashford, Diane Williams, and Pat Connolly; sports medicine experts such as Dr. Charles Yesalis of Penn State (who has become a friend and collaborator); and college football coaches such as Joe Paterno and Bo Schembechler. I too got a chance to speak.

By this time I had become one of the more vocal and visible personalities on this issue. I had already given dozens (today, the number is closer to hundreds) of talks at schools and colleges, coaches' and trainers' groups, even medical conventions. Some called me a fanatic, a flake, a nuisance (whenever there was an inaccuracy in a story, I would dash off a letter to the offender—I might have written up to five or six a week). Others recognized that I had extensive firsthand experience and had become quite knowledgeable on the subject.

All who spoke before the committee advocated passage of the legislation and, of course, spoke out against steroid use, and eventually the bill was passed. But the initial report contained a number of errors of fact and judgment. It stated: "In sum, the evidence is overwhelming: steroids are dangerous drugs that can permanently disfigure their young users—and, too often, take their young lives."

That is completely false. Thus far, in roughly four decades there have been five documented deaths, out of perhaps three million users. That's hardly "overwhelming." The report also mentions "physical dependence." There has yet been no medical evidence to bolster the contention that steroids are physically addictive; it just isn't so. (In the final report, after consultations with Dr. Charles Yesalis, corrections were made.)

In using scare tactics to push through a good bill, some would contend that it's just good politics. But is that necessary? Must the truth be bent to straighten out a bad situation? Are we such a passive people that we need to be scared, lied, or manipulated into doing the right thing?

There is enough evidence on the *possible* dangers of androgenic-anabolic steroids—certainly enough "scientific" speculation—to suffice. It certainly is dangerous for young people to be taking steroids. The drugs can seal their bone plates and stunt their growth. And it's possible that when all the studies are in, the truth will be even more frightening than we currently know. But right now we just don't have all the facts.

Other disappointments involving this bill related to the testimony of Pete Rozelle and, especially, Chuck Noll.

I expected nothing more from Commissioner P.R. than the 20 minutes of puffball he so sincerely pitched. In Rozelle's rambling opening statement, with his lawyer at his side, he offered little evidence that the NFL, in his illustrious 29-year term, had done anything more to curtail the steroid scourge than distribute a short educational film to high schools in 1987–88; it was almost sad as he mentioned this one fact in great detail.

Two months before testifying at this hearing, Pete Rozelle had sent a letter to NFL players advising them of a shift from a non-punitive to a punitive drug policy. Rozelle wrote, "(1) that steroids can give a competitive advantage to athletes that use them; (2) that steroid use may increase the risk of injuries both to the user and to other players; and (3) that steroids may result in other very significant health risks, both in the short run and in years to come."

Would that not seem slightly contradictory in light of Rozelle's reply to Senator Biden's question on whether there would be a decrease in player size if steroids were eliminated from pro football (as Bobby Beathard, now the general manager of the San Diego Chargers, had contended)?

"I really don't think so," Rozelle said. "I don't feel

[steroids] are that much of a benefit, and I don't think the size would be that reduced.

"In other words," he continued, "you can achieve the same thing through more wholesome means: exercise and vitamins and so forth."

(Which is it, Commissioner: "competitive advantage" or not "much of a benefit"?)

Before Chuck Noll's turn at the mike, Senator Biden alluded to the fact that the "distinguished witness" was the "second winningest coach, I need not tell you, in NFL history and the only coach in the NFL to have won four Super Bowl Championships." Senator Biden then thanked Chuck for a great "personal favor"—sending autographed Steeler footballs to the senator's two sons, who were hospitalized after an accident that killed their mother and sister. While I certainly commend Chuck for that thoughtful gesture, I perceived many of his comments that day to be extremely thoughtless and hypocritical.

"I think [steroid use] came into professional football from Olympic weight lifters and coaches and has grown from small dosages to mega-doses in pursuit of mega-bucks," Chuck said in his opening remarks.

Typical. Blame the players for their greed, while ignoring any part that the coaches or the league may have played in perpetuating this problem.

"[Steroid use] produces a 'rather be in the weight room, rather look at myself in the mirror,' than a person who wants to be successful on the football field," Chuck said. And he added: "Steroids, although they provide weight room strength, do not provide playing strength."

Both statements are complete folly, and I would think Chuck knows it. Speaking for myself and many of the other men who took steroids while playing for Chuck Noll, none of us used the drugs for any other reason than to become better football players. For us, they were vocational—not recreational—drugs. We didn't use them to look good at the beach or to win bodybuilding contests. We used them to become more productive at our jobs, and as long as we performed competently—and four Super Bowl rings attest to some level of football competence—the coaches never had a problem. The only time I was ever criticized for steroid use was when the drugs may have contributed to my muscle injuries.

As I've mentioned, on at least one occasion after I pulled a hamstring, Chuck angrily castigated me—justifiably—for my juice use contributing to an increased susceptibility to injury. If Chuck was so ignorant about the use of these drugs, as he indicated elsewhere in his testimony, how could he be aware of such a key piece of information relating to their effects?

The committee actually did press Chuck on one issue, that of extraordinary weight gains in a relatively short time—citing experts' testimony that it would be "virtually impossible for anyone to add 25 pounds of muscle mass no matter what they did . . . within a year period" without chemical enhancement.

Chuck said then that "there have been, and I know for a fact, people will put on that kind of weight from one season to the other because they have trained in the past, and it isn't over a one-year period of time but rather the backlog or the years of training allow them to do this."

Perhaps Chuck figured that if he said something authoritatively (and yet fuzzily) enough, people would buy it. But that is total bushwah, and Chuck is too smart not to know it. I, too, personally know lots of people who have gained a lot of weight in a short time, but that's from eating, and most of it is fat. No one can gain great amounts—20, 25, or 30 pounds—of sheer muscle weight (especially in a short time) without using some chemical component. And I, for one, would like to meet those medical marvels that apparently only Chuck has known.

"It is counterproductive to be dependent on the pill or to think you can get something out of a bottle," Chuck said in his testimony. "When we sign a player, we sign a whole person. We get the whole package, his physical makeup as well as his mental and emotional state, his fears, his hangups, his beliefs, and his addictions."

Not to impugn the integrity of Chuck or several of his recent draft picks, but what kind of package does one get with players who are known steroid users? Both Tom Ricketts, the Steelers' first-round pick in 1989, and Craig Veasey, the team's 1990 third-round choice, tested positive for steroids *before* they were drafted.

But perhaps the biggest misstatement of all concerned the matter of painkillers. Senator Biden posed the question:

"There are those who suggested that there is a mentality among team doctors that killing pain is an important function of a team physician, as you want those folks to be able to play. And the reason for the steroid mentality, to the extent that it exists among players, is not somehow disassociated from the notion of killing pain. If an athlete has a serious muscle pull, or a problem with his shoulder, the team doctor will shoot him up, and he will be able to play this game." Finally, Biden asked the question, "Is that fact or fiction?"

"From our standpoint," Chuck responded, "that is fiction. Pain is analyzed to a great deal of, you know, our doctors, what is the pain there? Let me put it that way. I am not saying that shots for pain have not been given, but they are not given just to get rid of pain.

"If pain is there indicating that someone should not play, then he is not going to play. If killing the pain will cause further injury, then it is not the way we want to go. If it is something that is minor, then that is done. But pain killing just for that is not done."

I looked at Bill Fralic, who was sitting next to me in the hearing room, and we both smiled. Virtually every pro football player at one time or another has taken or has been asked to take the needle that would enable him to play through the pain. In fact, I remembered numerous times with the Steelers when Chuck Noll told hurt players that the team physician could block off their pain without risking further injury. In typically sick locker room humor, we dubbed those players who agreed to take the needle members of the "Block Party." (Gary Dunn, perhaps the "sickest" of us all, used to personally observe these weekly painkilling sessions, whether he needed a shot or not. When I asked him about it, he just shrugged and said, "I like to watch.")

Senator Biden followed up with another question to Chuck: "The fact that pain killers are there does not put great pressure on the player to say, go ahead, Doc, give me the shot, and give a rationale for why the shot should be given?"

"You know, in my experience, I do not think we have ever had anybody do that," Chuck said. "When there is pain, and I am sure everybody in this room has experienced pain of some sort, it is there for a reason and you want to know the reason why. If there is a good explanation for why it is there, and if it is saying do not play, you do not play."

Chuck may have been able to bamboozle some politicians in rep ties and tailored jackets, but every man who's ever suited up in faceguards and pads must have chortled at the naïveté of anyone who bought this line of self-serving bull.

Prior to the hearings I had faxed a nine-page statement to the committee. Then, after I had arrived in some physical discomfort—weakened from the medication, and advised by my doctor not to travel—I was told that I'd have but five minutes to make my points. I would have crawled from Pittsburgh to Washington to speak for five seconds that day.

When I first was diagnosed with cardiomyopathy, I felt helpless and depressed. It was not something that I could fix in the weight room. And so, to give some purpose to my life, it became my mission to learn about the possible dangers of steroids, while also clamoring for more research.

Thinking about the subject, finding out about it, and, finally, helping to educate others—especially young people—was like lifting a weight *off* of my shoulders. It gave me reason to get out of bed each morning.

In my allotted five minutes, I addressed the steady escalation of a "chemical war" in professional football. Contrary to Chuck Noll's previous remarks, weight training had become an accepted, effective way to increase strength (and increase football skills). One of the most productive methods of weight training—the "secret within a secret"—was the use of anabolic-androgenic steroids.

I told of the drugs' genesis in this country (see Chapter 9) and how and when they seeped into professional football (most likely in 1963, with the Chargers). And of course I spoke of the need for education—a national research center, perhaps in cooperation with the National Institutes of Health. The Soviets, I mentioned, have been doing research since the fifties; might not some interactive *glasnost* help counter our own ignorance on the subject?

What I did not have time to address that day (though my opinions had been faxed to Senator Biden earlier) were the ignorance and ineptitude on the part of Pete Rozelle's NFL stewardship in dealing with the steroid issue (which I'll address at length in Chapter 11).

You can fool *some* of the people some of the time . . .

I've always been driven—as a football player, as a weight-lifter, and even as a steroid user. And now, since my time may be short, I feel even more compelled to get out there and change people's minds.

Some things I cannot change. I certainly can't stop some folks from believing that I'm an unfit transplant candidate. Or a flake. Those beliefs, and those people, are outside my control. It won't, however, stop me from trying.

9

STEROIDS—AN HISTORICAL, MEDICAL, AND SOCIOLOGICAL OVERVIEW

HISTORY

THE ANCIENT GREEKS, those fabled Olympians, were not the purists we once imagined. Many of them used a number of supposedly performance-enhancing substances to get a leg (arm, foot, etc.) up on the competition. Wrestlers reputedly racked up megadoses of lamb—up to ten pounds a day—in order to stack up on protein. Distance runners chewed tons of sesame seeds in the belief that they increased endurance. Other competitors drank wine mixed with strychnine and/ or hallucinogenic mushrooms to help psych themselves up for their events.

Greek wrestlers, boxers, distance runners, and discuss throwers were reportedly paid today's equivalent of $900,000 in order to compete in ye old Games. Officials were also bribed. Cheaters were punished in a novel, yet indelible, way. Those caught soiling the Olympic ideal had their names, along with their family trees, etched in infamy onto the marble pedestals, or zanes, that fronted the Olympic stadium. (Apparently the pristine appearance of some of our venerated institutions was also largely a myth. In the nineteenth century, two of the United States' most prestigious academic institutions, Harvard and Yale, wrote the book on cheating in college athletics, with payments to ringers as well as bribes to competitiors and officials.)

Steroids did not appear until around the first third of the twentieth century.

In 1935, Charles D. Kochakian, a researcher from the University of Rochester, was credited with chemically identifying the male sex hormone, testosterone. Four years later, Dr. Ove Boje theorized that the administration of sex hormones might increase physical output and performance. Boje was also the first to warn athletes of AAS's potential health effects, stating that steroid use "should definitely be avoided, since it may involve dangers the extent of which cannot be entirely gauged."

The first nonmedical uses of AAS occurred in World War II, during which, according to some accounts, German troops took steroids before battle in order to enhance aggressiveness and reduce their fear of violence. These reports are to be accepted skeptically, since there has been no mention of AAS usage in an examination of the records of Dr. Morrell, Adolf Hitler's quack physician.

Documented steroid use did occur after the war ended: emaciated, diseased victims of Hitler's monstrous concentration camps were given substantial doses of AAS for their potential protein and muscle-building properties.

According to well-documented evidence, the first athletes to exploit the use of AAS for a specific sporting edge were the Soviet weightlifters of the forties and fifties. In the 1954 World Games in Vienna, U.S. weightlifting team physician Dr. John Ziegler was told by his Russian counterpart that the Soviet athletes were using testosterone.

The Soviets, as usual, dominated the competition, and Dr. Ziegler returned home to York, Pennsylvania, where he began experimenting with various dosages of testosterone on himself and several weightlifters at the York Barbell Club. He then was involved with Ciba Pharmaceuticals in creating the first American steroid, Dianabol (methandrostenolone), in 1958.

The word—and the drugs—soon spread in and around weightlifters and strength athletes; by the mid-sixties, some of the top-ranked track and field stars had taken steroids, including Randy Matson (who used them while preparing for the 1964 Olympics), Dallas Long, Hal Connolly, Bill Toomey, and Russ Hodge.

At the 1968 Olympic Games in Mexico City—best known for the controversial black-power salutes raised by a couple of American sprinters—there was little debate regarding the morality or propriety of performance-enhancing drugs. The only discussion was over which drug was the most effective, and what kind of amphetamines could go undetected in the then-primitive screening methods. (The first drug tests, primarily for amphetamines, were administered in 1965, precipitated by the deaths of several European cyclists. Anabolic-androgenic steroids weren't made a banned substance in Olympic competition until 1975, and the first test for AAS use was in Montreal in 1976.)

Bill Toomey, gold medalist in the decathlon in the '68 Olympics and winner of the prestigious Sullivan Award for outstanding amateur athlete of that year, later admitted that he had taken AAS to aid his performance. He hadn't planned on using any drugs for unfair advantage, he said, but soon found that most of his fellow competitors were using them; he then decided not to compete at an unfair disadvantage.

George Frenn, an American Olympic hammer thrower, said: "I think the bottom line is this: An athlete doesn't want to lose; but if he does, he wants to know that he was beaten by someone who is free of drugs."

At the 1970 World Weightlifting Championships in Columbus, Ohio, nine of the top 12 medalists were disqualified because urine tests had revealed amphetamine usage.

Ken Patera, an American lifter, called the action "ridiculous." Weightlifters, he said, had been using speed for years. Right after winning the 1971 Pan Am Games in Cali, Colombia, Patera looked forward to his matchup with the great Russian superheavyweight, Vassili Alexeev, in the upcoming '72 Olympics in Munich.

"Last year," Patera said, "the only difference between me and [Alexeev] was that I couldn't afford his drug bill. When I hit Munich, I'll weigh in at about 340, or maybe 350. Then, we'll see which are better—his steroids or mine."

The Russians had the better juice that year, winning gold medals in the lightweight, heavyweight, and superheavyweight (Alexeev) categories; all but one of the other six weight classes were won by Eastern Bloc athletes.

After the success of the East German women swimmers at the 1976 Olympics at Montreal, their coach was asked why so many of the women had deep voices. He replied: "We have come here to swim, not to sing."

The fact is that Eastern Bloc athletes have always been pioneers—some might call them guinea pigs—when it came to chemical experimentation in the world of sports. But winning in that world often came at a very high price.

When René Vogel, one of those East German swimmers, defected to the West in 1979, she described a system of sports camps where children were fed steroids as early as 10 years old. "I honestly cannot name one [athlete]—and I know just about all of them personally—who is not using some [steroid]," she said.

For years there have been whispers of early deaths of

Soviet athletes—59 over the past three decades, according to one source, who died before the age of 45.

In the United States, we have yet to accurately assess the usage—or the damage—of anabolic-androgenic steroids by our athletes. But certain figures are undeniable. The average weight of a college football lineman in 1949 was 195 pounds; forty years later, it was 257 pounds. In 1989, there were more than 15 offensive lines in colleges football that averaged more than 290 pounds.

Where did this newfound bulk come from? Wheaties?

In 1987, the first nationwide study of AAS use by American high school students was conducted at Penn State by Doctors Charles Yesalis and William Buckley. They found that 6.6 percent of male high school seniors—approximately 250,000 young men—reported some use. While that number was surprising enough, there were even more shocking results: nearly 40 percent of the users reported completing five or more cycles (I didn't do five cycles until my fifth year in the pros); 44 percent "stacked" steroids (took two or more kinds); 38 percent used injectables; 38 percent had initiated use before the age of 16; and more than one third of the users did not even participate in sports.

Furthermore, the majority of these young AAS users perceived their relative strength to be greater than average and assessed their health as very good or better; their self-perceptions were generally more extreme than the nonusers'. The study also indicated that 40 percent of this group did not want AAS use stopped in sports, even if their competitors did not take them. One in four of the self-reported users stated their intentions to continue taking AAS even at the risk of dire health consequences such as sterility, heart attacks, or liver cancer. This study concluded that a total of approximately 500,000 teenagers are using or have used anabolic-androgenic steroids.

In 1989, the state of Michigan produced a study that said 27,000 teenagers in the state were using steroids.

The Department of Health and Human Services presented a report in 1990 that estimated 250,000 adolescents were taking AAS. Detailed interviews with 55 adolescent users revealed that two thirds of the kids believed that their coaches did not disapprove of their use; half thought that their parents were aware of their use; and 82 percent did not believe that there were long-term health dangers. (Other telling stats: 86 percent used AAS for improved appearance; 93 percent believed their AAS use was a "good" decision; 89 percent increased their dosage over time; 72 percent stacked the drugs; 25 percent sold drugs to support their "habit"; and 86 percent had no intention of stopping their AAS use.)

Additionally, there is anedotal information of sixth grade taking steroids—11, and 12-year olds.

Compare the above statistics to a poll of high school coaches conducted by *USA Today* in 1990, in which only one percent believed that AAS use was a problem. What then *does* constitute a problem?

One wonders what is the coaches' problem if they cannot, or refuse to, see something that has grown to such enormous proportions.

MEDICAL (AND PSYCHOLOGICAL) PROPERTIES

There are two basic kinds of anabolic-androgenic steroids: orals and injectables. All steroids, which are derived from the male hormone testosterone, contain anabolic and androgenic properties (most have more of one than the other). The anabolic (tissue-building) component helps build muscle tissue, while the androgenic (masculinizing) characteristic comes from the influence of the male sex hormone testosterone in the drug.

The three subclassifications of AAS are: testosterone esters (these theoretically affect the internal organs less than the other groups, which is one reason why they're used); nore-testosterone esters (which are more easily detectable); and 17-alkalated compounds (which can be toxic to the liver).

Much of the debate over the effectiveness of AAS in athletics was, until 1984, linked to the then-twenty-five existing studies in the literature. Approximately half of these studies indicated definite strength and size gains, while the other half did not. In 1984, Herbert Haupt and George Rovere's definitive review of this literature for *The American Journal of Sports Medicine* concluded that inconsistent study protocols revealed inconsistent study yield. In essence, the poorly designed studies, which did not find efficacy of AAS use, did not use trained athletes in proper conditions with adequate diets.

The benefits of AAS use in athletics are now well-documented: increased lean body mass and strength (which usually translates into increased overall athletic performance), as well as perhaps its most underrated aspect, increased recuperative properties (with which athletes are able to train harder and more frequently and make greater gains in shorter periods).

AAS's have been widely used for legitimate medical purposes: osteoporosis (a bone disease, in which steroids help recalcify bones); hypogonadism (testes don't produce testosterone); burn patients, to faciliate recovery; cancer and other patients, recuperating from surgery; certain blood disorders (such as anemia); and, in a recently completed test study, for use as a possible male contraceptive.

For those using the drugs to bulk up for athletics, one of

the short-term liabilities is the increased likelihood of injuries. The human body is designed to carry a natural muscle mass. When you chemically engineer a newer, larger physique, you're putting on more bulk than the frame can handle. Connective tissues—ligaments, muscles, tendons—can become more brittle, and more suspectible to injuries.

Of course, the catch-22 in contact sports such as football is that if you don't bulk up with AAS, you're more likely to get injured by guys who, being twice as big and fast, may have.

The androgenic component, in particular, seems to lend itself to more muscle tightness and proneness to injury. With steroids that have more of the anabolic tissue-building properties, there is not the same suceptibility to injury (although they are reputedly more likely to adversely affect the internal organs).

So choose your potion: highly androgenic steroids such as Anadrol, Halotestin, or one of the testosterone esters; or particularly anabolic drugs such as Primabolin, Anavar, or Deca-Durabolin (the latter in particular reduces the likelihood of muscle pulls, yet is probably the most easily detectable since it stays in the system longer).

The long-term health effects on the individual are unknown. Thus far, the fatal incidents ascribed to AAS use have been few (a total of five documented deaths).

Dr. Karl Friedl, one of the most respected scientists in the field, published a recent report for the National Institute on Drug Abuse (NIDA) on AAS abuse. In the cases of significant morbidity or mortality in athletes associated with AAS use, Friedl states that:

> a common aspect of these athlete case reports is the inadequate description of their drug use. More pointedly, in

*each of the four cases resulting in death [another fatality
was discovered after the study], use of androgens appear
to be a chance discovery which gave the case report
current relevance. . . . Other athletes with significant
morbidity may conceal their drug use when complications
arise. . . . No systematic study of the medical risks of
androgen use by any athletes has ever been conducted and
even the population of adult athletes at risk remains unde-
fined.*

The cardiovascular system in particular may be at risk
with the sustained, significant use of AAS (excepting testosterone esters). The drugs seems to alter blood lipid
(cholesterol) profiles by raising LDL (low-density lipids), the
"bad" cholesterol, while reducing HDL (high-density lipids), the "good" cholesterol. So by cycling steroids over a
long period of time, theoretically the user could be a prime
candidate for atherosclerosis—the most common heart disease, often associated with a high-fat, high-LDL diet. Larry
Pacifico, a former world-champion powerlifter, has blamed
his atherosclerosis on extensive AAS use. I'm not familiar
with the details of his case, especially the nature of his
other drug or alcohol history, so I can't comment on it
further.

Other possible long-term health effects of anabolic-
androgenic steroids include platelet aggregation in the
blood, which enhances risk of stroke, and liver disease.
Some medical experts maintain that massive doses of
steroids affect the liver similarly to the way alcohol beats
up on the organ, making it more susceptible to disease. Oral
steroids are cited as doubly threatening since they pass
through the liver twice—via the digestive tract and the
bloodstream. However, thus far there has been a low
incidence of *recorded* liver disease in AAS users.

The following short-term health effects are those that are

most frequently and universally associated with anabolic-
androgenic steroids.

In men: reduced sperm count; enlarged prostate; development of female-type breasts—gynecomastia—crassly referred to as "bitch tits."

In women: deepening of voice; increased facial and body
hair; pectoral enlargement (not breast enlargement). Other
studies indicate more severe problems, including possible
sterility (although as yet there are no documented cases).

In children: growth can be stunted.

For both men and women: acne, greasy hair; scalp hair
loss; increased body hair; increased number of headaches;
increased irritability or aggression; depression; sleepless-
ness; euphoria; increased sex drive; decreased sex drive;
fluid retention; increased urine output; muscle spasms;
elevated liver enzymes; shrunked testes.

Most of the short-term effect of AAS—similar to those of
male puberty (since all anabolic steroids are synthetic
forms of testosterone, it's no coincidence)—are transitory.
Yet in some instances the individual's body shape and size
can change permanently. As the AAS-faciliated cells en-
large, so do the myofibrils (micro muscle fibers). And it
appears that a portion of this enlargement is irreversible.

Soon after a cycle is completed, there is usually a significant reduction in weight, most of which is water, but
much of the muscle mass remains. (After my first, and only,
cycle as a college sophomore, I gained thirty pounds in six
weeks; I basically maintained that weight for my entire
collegiate career. Before entering the pros, when I wanted to
become bigger, I had to cycle again.)

Certainly the effectiveness of AAS depends on one's
genetic makeup and metabolism; everyone is different.
Usually, if someone is 5'1" and 120 pounds, he can only get
so big, whereas an individual who is 6'1" and 230 pounds

could probably derive much greater applicable gains. The bigger the frame, the more meat you can ultimately hang on it.

Some of you technical types might want to know how steroids are synthesized into protein at the cellular level. In clinical terms, here's how: Steroid hormones are secreted through the blood after being synthesized in the glands. Eventually the steroid hormone binds to the nucleus of the cell, which is considered the target organ for that particular hormone. When the intracellular steroid/receptor complex is in the cell nucleus and binds with the nuclear DNA, then the mechanics of transcription are enhanced.

Out of this process, messenger RNA is formed and free to leave the nucleus. Then messenger RNA binds to ribosomal RNA from the cytoplasm of the cell, and the translation of messenger RNA takes place, allowing protein synthesis to occur in the golgi apparatus of the cell. The kind of alteration the steroid hormone exerts on the cell determines the type of cellular protein formed. In the case of testosterone and skeletal muscle cells, steroid-increased hormone regulation usually results in increased protein as well as increased muscle size and strength as a group, of which the individual cell is a part. Increased individual muscle size and strength contribute to the whole.

In short, when proper diet and training are tacked onto this cellular process, the skeletal muscle is going to grow. And grow.

I want to clarify this point: One *can* get bigger and stronger in a well-designed program without the use of drugs. But not *as* big and *as* strong.

As far as we now know, steroids are not physically addictive. But there does seem to be a strong potential for psychological dependence. As your body gets more yoked and roped (muscularly defined), there is more positive reinforcement from one's peers and even more reinforcement from society ("bigger is better . . .").

To press that point: Most élite athletes stop AAS usage only when their competitive careers end. In the meantime, many of the former 98-pound weaklings will continue to use the drugs even after the desired results are attained; the individual's self-worth often becomes tied into his or her improved physical appearance, and there is a dependence on the "magic" formula that has made it happen.

Another indicator of possible psychological addiction is that rarely do you see AAS users do just one cycle; they become hooked on the results and the possibilities of these drugs.

One of the biggest psychological problems with anabolic-androgenic steroids is denial. This was confirmed in a study of élite powerlifters done by Dr. Yesalis in which only 55 percent acknowledged steroid use (in a population with a nearly 100 percent perceived involvement). Many top athletes would sooner admit that they snorted coke for fun than acknowledge their AAS usage; they often refuse to recognize that their performances may have been in some way improved by artificial means.

Some recent preliminary studies have indicated effects of AAS on the receptor sites in the brain—in short, the possibility that one's wires can be permanently jostled or crossed (leading, perhaps, to an increased susceptibility to aggression and hostility).

The fact that these drugs can raise the level of aggressiveness is perceived by many athletics as a distinct asset. I would note, however, that overly aggressive behavior is not suddenly precipitated in someone who's essentially even-tempered. The so-called 'roid "attacks" may even be misleading; anecdotal evidence indicates that only people with a predisposition to violence experience extreme rages or psychotic breaks.

When we talk of performance-enhancing drugs, anabolic-androgenic steroids get all the press (and glamor), but they're only a small part of the problem.

The human growth hormone (HGH) is becoming increasingly popular among strength athletes—either in its pure form as a cellular extract (from cadavers) or, more commonly, as a synthetic drug such as Protropin, which has many of the anabolic properties of steroids and is also undetectable in drug tests. (There are also growth hormone releasers or stimulators such as L-Dopa, clonidine, and propranolol.)

Protropin is another example of how a drug developed for a specific medical purpose—its original use was for children suffering from dwarfism—has been subverted by people looking for a sporting advantage. (There's additional controversy swirling around the drug's manufacturer, Genentech Inc., which some have accused of trying to market the drug without sufficient cause to small children in the possibility that it *might* help them grow.)

While we don't know all the long-term side effects of most steroids, we do know at least one of HGH: acromegaly. (Both André the Giant, the wrestler, and actor Richard Kiel, "Jaws" in James Bond movies, are acromegalics—those who have abnormally elevated levels of growth hormone—which often means heart disease and a short life span.) If you see bodybuilders with protruding brows and lantern jaws, they're probably using megadoses of HGH. It's also rapidly becoming the drug of choice for top women bodybuilders because it has the anabolic, fat-mobilizing properties of steroids without the masculinizing side effects.

Former NFL defensive lineman Lyle Alzado has blamed his brain cancer on megadoses of HGH, taken during his unsuccessful comeback attempt in 1990. Alzado also admitted to using anabolic-androgenic steroids virtually non-stop for more than 20 years.

Al Oerter, the great Olympic discus thrower, once said that some athletes would "devour a Brillo pad" if it would improve their performance. I probably would have. But I never took HGH for two basic reasons: I didn't know that much about the drug (it was still relatively new during the peak of my usage); and the possibility of looking like an acromegalic was never that appealing.

When I was in powerlifting, people would take anything and everything (with the possible exception of a Brillo pad) to give themselves an edge: coke and methedrine, to get that big surge prior to a big lift; methyl-testosterone, and AAS that also generates temporary explosiveness; even rhesus monkey hormones (for who knows what reason). I've also heard of lifters injecting pure adrenaline into their system, which is pure insanity.

I personally know bodybuilders who've stacked eight to 12 steroids at a time while supplementing them with HGH, HGH stimulators, amphetamines, and diuretics (to reduce water weight and make the physique look more "cut" on the day of the contest). Other body "cutting" techniques— to get that "peeled" or "inside out" look so appealing to judges—are to use thyroid hormones to help thin the skin; and Wyadase, normally a spreading solution for oil-based drugs, which is used a "spot reducer"—that is, injected directly into the area that one wants reduced or tightened.

There is no end to the means that competitors will go in order to succeed. Some have gone too far. Over a period of four years (1986–90), 18 European cyclists died "mysteriously," their deaths linked to a single performance-enhancing drug: recombinant erythropoietin (EPO).

EPO, a genetically engineered drug created for people

suffering from kidney failure, increases red blood cells; this is especially appealing to endurance athletes since the increase in red cells then increases the body's ability to carry oxygen. In a study conducted by the Stockholm Institute of Gymnastics and Sports, an individual's aerobic performance improved 10 percent after use of the drug.

The downside is that EPO thickens the blood, which becomes even more concentrated as dehydration occurs during the course of a race. "Pretty soon you have mud instead of blood," said Dr. Randy Eichner, chief of hematology at the University of Oklahoma. "Then you have trouble." The thick, sticky blood can cause "clotting, stroke or heart failure."

Since EPO is a model of a naturally occurring protein, it is also undetectable in any drug test. So the real mystery is not how these cyclists died; it is why athletes are so eager to take a drug that they know could kill them.

SOCIOLOGICAL EFFECTS

Virtually every day there's a story about athletes using performance-enhancing drugs. The situation is so endemic— it may be closer to an *epidemic*—that the innumerable accounts probably don't even register on the average reader or viewer. Here's a short list of steroid-related items that appeared in the media over the course of about 18 months.

JANUARY 1990: In an investigative report, Washington D.C. TV station WJLA accuses Dr. Forest Tennant, then NFL drug advisor, of covering up the positive cocaine tests of three white quarterbacks.

FEBRUARY 1990: In a follow-up on Dr. Tennant, WSLA reports that the NFL drug "czar" falsified drug tests of NASCAR driver Tim Richmond.

FEBRUARY 1990: Police find 400 hypodermic needles in the possession of New York Jets reserve linebacker Joe Mott, but he denies using the needles for any drugs, including steroids.

FEBRUARY 1990: Craig Veasey, the Steelers third-round draft choice who tested positive for steroids, says he used the drugs to "heal an injured wrist and run faster." Chuck Noll says: "It wasn't a long-term thing. . . . I'm satisfied with his story."

MARCH 1990: *The National* reports the wasted physical condition of pro wrestler Superstar Billy Graham, whose doctors directly cite steroids as the cause of hip replacement surgery, as well as the need for several more major surgeries on his back and legs (including possible amputation of both legs). Graham says 90 percent of pro wrestlers abuse steroids.

MARCH 1990: The *Detroit News* reports that seven Michigan State players took steroids prior to the 1987 Rose Bowl. Tony Mandarich, Green Bay Packers offensive tackle, is cited as the players' "doctor/mentor."

APRIL 1990: Tampa Bay Buccaneers offensive lineman Carl Bax is indicted for possession of anabolic steroids with intent to distribute.

MAY 1990: John Armond De Fendis, former U.S. bodybuilding champ, is arrested for importing $20,000 worth of anabolic steroids from France.

AUGUST 1990: Former Notre Dame football player Steve Huffman says in *Sports Illustrated* that head coach Lou Holtz knew about AAS use on the Irish team, and that two assistant coaches urged him (Huffman) to use them.

SEPTEMBER 1990: Former Oklahoma coach Barry Switzer admits in *The National* that he was aware some of his players were taking steroids but did not confront the users. "[Steroid use] had been going on for years and no one cared because no one was getting hurt," he says. "You're not robbing 7-Elevens; you're not murdering someone to get steroids. No coach said, 'Go take steroids.' But I knew if a kid pumped himself up [and] came back over the summer. I said, 'That kid's got to be on steroids.' Today, we test."

SEPTEMBER 1990: *USA Today* reports that for the first time in its twenty-six-year history, competitors in this year's Mr. Olympia bodybuilding contest will be tested for "muscle-building drugs."

FALL 1990: Matthew Dufresne, reigning Mr. Universe, is indicted on federal charges of conspiring to smuggle anabolic steroids into the United States.

OCTOBER 1990: In Dr. Robert Voy's book, *Drugs, Sport, and Politics*, the former chief medical officer for the USOC contends that some athletes are being warned in advance of their weekly "random" tests; he claims that 50 percent of U.S. Olympic athletes use drugs. Voy says that the sport of track, supervised by the International Amateur Athletic Federation (IAAF), has the "darkest history when it comes to drug abuse among athletes— and the unwillingness of officials to work effectively toward eliminating the problem." Voy also accuses the IAAF of drug "cover-ups."

OCTOBER 1990: Randy Barnes and Butch Reynolds, world record-holders in the shot put and 400-meter run, respectively, test positive for steroids (Barnes for methyl-testosterone) and are suspended for two years (through the '92 Summer Olympics).

DECEMBER 1990: Dr. Charles Yesalis of Penn State, in conjunction with researchers at five other universities, releases a study which estimates that 14.7 percent of male and 5.9 percent of female college athletes use steroids (29 percent of college football players).

DECEMBER 1990: In a news conference to promote his return to international competition after a two-year-ban, sprinter Ben Johnson says that he's "glad" he tested positive for steroids in the '88 Olympics. "My health is the most important thing," he says. "I want to have children, get married. . . . If I had kept taking [steroids], I could have had side effects with my liver. I'm very glad I got caught. Everything happens for a reason."

JANUARY 1991: In his book *Speed Trap*, Ben Johnson's former coach, Charlie Francis, details Ben's drug use—and seven years of beating drug tests—while maintaining that most world-class runners also take steroids. "I don't call it cheating," says Francis. "My definition of cheating is something that nobody else is doing."

APRIL 1991: The *Los Angeles Times* breaks a story on USC football players using substitute urine to circumvent drug testing.

MAY 1991: *USA Today* reports that the NCAA's new (since August 1990) program of year-round, spot-checking AAS testing "appears to have cut down on college football players' use of anabolic steroids."

MAY 1991: The San Francisco 49ers sign shotputter Randy Barnes, serving a two-year track and field suspension for steroid use (see above), to an NFL contract.

JUNE 1991: Dr. Jamie Astaphan, Ben Johnson's former physician, is suspended from practicing medicine for eighteen months and fined $5,000 by a panel of four doctors from the College of Physicians and Surgeons of Ontario. Astaphan argued that he had prescribed steroids for Johnson and other sprinters out of fear that they would "kill themselves" if they continued to administer their own treatments.

JUNE 1991: Butch Reynolds, also on a two-year track and field suspension for steroid use (see above), is temporarily reinstated on appeal. He continues to proclaim his innocence, blaming faulty testing procedures. "I don't take steroids," he says. "I [want] them to take out my liver, do anything they [want] to do to prove that."

JUNE 1991: Hulk Hogan, Roddy Piper, and three other professional wrestlers are cited as patients of Dr. George Zahorian III, who is convicted in a Harrisburg, Pennsylvania, court of illegally prescribing steroids (the wrestlers are not charged).

JUNE 1991: Lyle Alzado, former NFL defensive lineman, blames his rare form of brain cancer on his extensive steroid use. He believes that human growth hormone, in particular, adversely affected his immune system.

JULY 1991: In what is called the largest AAS bust ever, thirty-three people, including redshirted Arizona State football player Robert W. "Bill" Doverspike, are arrested. Doverspike reportedly told the arresting officers that he provided his teammates with steroids. ASU's associate athletic director Herman Frazier says: "Our athletes were tested [for steroids] by the NCAA in the spring, and we had no positives." He adds, "I don't feel it's a problem at this time."

steroids. ASU's associate athletic director Herman Frazier says: "Our athletes were tested [for steroids] by the NCAA in the spring, and we had no positives." He adds, "I don't feel it's a problem at this time."

JULY 1991: Randy Barnes is cut by the San Francisco 49ers.

JULY 1991: Terry Long, offensive lineman for the Pittsburgh Steelers, is admitted to Allegheny General Hospital after a reported suicide attempt. The day before, he'd been notified by the NFL of his positive steroid test.

AUGUST 1991: In an interview on a Houston TV station (KTRK), former Steeler Ernie Holmes talks about the prevalence of drugs during his playing days: "I found a ready supply of acid, speed, whatever you might need to get up for a game." He adds: "I know Steelers who were using steroids. I could name names, but certain individuals wouldn't want their names called."

10

STEROIDS—
THE HITS AND MYTHS

WE ARE CURRENTLY entering the fifth decade of AAS use and in the world of sports; in recent years, these drugs have advanced beyond powerlifting, bodybuilding, football, track and field, wrestling, swimming, cycling, marathon running—virtually every athletic arena with the exception of the Special Olympics—into the realm of entertainment, law enforcement, firefighting, and so on.

In short, anabolic-androgenic steroids have become almost as much a part of our culture as fast food and instant photography—except, as I've tried to emphasize, steroids are not shortcuts to a quick fix.

Nor are they likely to wreak the sort of devastating effects that some have threatened. It's ironic that the same people who were claiming steroids were a placebo just a few years ago are now blaming these same drugs with causing "liver and bone damage, disturbances in metabolic and sexual functions, and, among women, virilization and menstrual upset" (from a recent booklet, "Doping," put out by the International Olympic Committee medical commission).

How can testosterone enanthate be called a dangerous drug when the World Health Organization (WHO) recently cited it as a "safe, stable, effective and reversible" male contraceptive?

We can't have it both ways. Nor can we keep changing our minds about these drugs every few years. Soon there'll be other drugs that will surpass the ones we now have. The technology is changing by the minute. Our outlook is antiquated.

One benchmark commonly used to determine the danger of any drug is its toxicity level. Here's an interesting test: Line up bottles filled with aspirin, Darvon, amphetamines, and Dianabol. Suppose you were forced to swallow the contents of one entire bottle; which would you choose? If you picked Dianabol, you would experience some immediate minor stomach discomfort. Yet had you ingested any one of the others, the effects conceivably could have been fatal.

I'm not sure what conclusions can be drawn there, other than the usual: We need to do much more research to determine when and how these drugs are harmful.

I find myself in an unusual position. Many people know me as that "steroid guy" who's been very vocal in clamoring for more tests, studies, and research. Some folks automatically assume I'm *anti*-steroids. I don't know what that means. If you ask me if kids should be taking steroids, I would say, absolutely not. But if you ask me whether or not athletes should be using performance-enhancing drugs, I can only respond from a moral stance.

I believe that all athletes should compete purely and cleanly. But is that realistic in today's sporting world? Current athletes are faced with a Hobson's Choice: Take drugs and expose themselves to possible health risks, or compete at a disadvantage.

I was pleased to play a small role in the passage of the 1990 Steroid Trafficking Act. In general, I supported the bill—especially the section that requires secondary schools to include AAS in their substance-abuse programs. But I did warn Senator Biden about some of the drawbacks in the antitrafficking laws. By cutting off the available route between the athlete and his doctor, you open up the avenues to the black market. Kids are now going to be buying these drugs from unscrupulous drug dealers. Who knows what they'll be getting? There are no health organizations or physicians on the black market to check out the purity of each substance. With many of the drugs sold out there being counterfeit, some will be harmlessly fake, while others could be extremely dangerous.

My own solution, which is admittedly not a very popular one (nor, again, very pragmatic), would be to legalize—or, at least, to regulate, control, and decriminalize—all drugs. If you take out the crime, you take out the criminal element.

I want to be clear about this: I do not advocate the *use* of drugs. But I question the effectiveness of any form of prohibition. It didn't work with alcohol. Can society curb man's basic appetites with legislation? With the current Supreme Court veering off into dangerously antilibertarian waters, I don't think we should so easily abandon some of our hard-won freedoms. I believe that we need to treat all use and abuse of drugs as more of a medical than a criminal or punitive problem.

Penalties and so-called disciplinary methods cannot truly deal with such a complex medical and social issue. Punitive drug testing doesn't even come close to attacking the root of the problem. It's "Just Say No" with a little added punch— lip service with a bite.

Drug testing. Just the sound of it has an ominous,

1984-ish connotation. Some would say it's a necessary evil. Yet while these tests have begun creeping and seeping into the real world—particularly in the workplace—nowhere is it more scrutinized than in the realm of sports.

Before we get into the ethics, here's some history.

Dope detection as we know it today was initiated at the Tour of Britain cycle races in 1965 and at the Olympic Games in 1968. AAS testing began at the Olympics in 1976 (all tests were announced until the post-Ben Johnson furor; now the tests are supposedly random). If an athlete was caught using any of the known existing drugs, he or she was suspended and all medals were taken away. At the time, however, many of the athletes were using the testosterone esters, which was (and is) one of the Achilles heels of drug testing.

One problem: it wasn't until 1982 that they even had a test for testosterone. Another problem: the test is easily beatable. Since every male has testosterone in his body, the IOC and most of the sports federations have set a ceiling: six parts testosterone to one part epitestosterone. If you're over the ceiling, you've tested positive for testosterone doping.

But that ceiling is a joke. To allow for individual differences in testosterone levels, and so as not to falsely accuse anyone, it was set way too high. Instead, because many athletes have learned to manipulate the ratio by simply *adding* epitestosterone to their system, we're seeing a lot of false negatives. Most athletes know that the ceiling is too high, and they can theoretically take up to 300 milligrams of testosterone a week and still test clean. (A recent study by Karl Friedl, in which he administered to individuals dosages up to 300 milligrams of testosterone cypionate a week for six weeks, confirmed this theory.)

To ensure an acceptable ratio, many athletes are doing self-testing in "safe" laboratories. There's so much money at stake, it obviously pays to take these precautions. (There are even masking agents such as the mail-order product Defend that you take three hours before an announced test; supposedly it conceals almost any AAS from detection, with the exception of Deca-Durabolin.)

The announced test is, of course, one of the real flaws in the system. Since athletes and their coaches have become so sophisticated in manipulating or masking their drug use, you have to be really stupid or really, really unlucky to get caught. And again, except for Deca-Durabolin, virtually every other steroid is out of your system in one month.

Before the 1980 Games in Moscow, which the United States boycotted, the IOC tested 1,500 athletes; not one came up positive (which, if nothing else, affirms the superiority of the Eastern Bloc in blocking AAS use from detection). At the 1984 Olympics in Los Angeles, there were 1,510 analyses and 17 positives—a 1.1 percent yield—though, for reasons known to the IOC, only 10 athletes were sanctioned. In the Seoul Olympics in 1988, 30 out of 1,500 athletes tested positive for AAS use (2 percent), though, again, only 10 were sanctioned.

Only the most naïve bureaucrat would contend that no more than two percent of our world-class amateur athletes use steroids. (One of those bureaucrats, former United States Olympic Committee [USOC] chief medical officer Dr. Robert Voy, stated that the number of U.S. Olympic athletes using performance-enhancing drugs is closer to 50 percent.)

In the year leading to the 1984 Olympic Games, the USOC even had a monitored program of informal drug testing—perhaps so our athletes could avoid "embarrassment" at the Games. The USOC knew that steroids were being used; officials had to be concerned that no one would be disqualified at the Olympics. If an athlete's sample came up positive during these informal tests, there were no sanctions. Apparently it was just that, a test, and athletes could then do whatever they had to in order to get clean for the real deal.

In unannounced tests (with no punitive actions) at USOC-sponsored events in 1984–85, positive results were 50 percent—obviously a more accurate, if still low, indicator.

That's not to say that unannounced tests are infallible. They still can't catch the adept testosterone/epitestosterone manipulator, nor is there yet a test for the human growth hormone or EPO. Plus, if the drug is not on record in the library of banned substances, there is no test for it. They can only find what they already know.

Drug testing in sports has been most successful when aimed at performance-enhancing drugs that, in order to be most effective, need to be in the body at the time of competition. However, with drugs such as steroids that are primarily used during training periods, there is less precision in the screening process.

Random drug testing is obviously the most effective method of prohibition, although it is very costly (for example, it's estimated that it would now run about $100 million to test every high school football player in America). Recently, many of the sporting federations that had once used announced testing procedures—such as the USOC, the NCAA, the Athletic Congress (TAC) and the NFL— have adopted random drug testing.

The reliability of the tests, which has often been challenged, has also improved. Most screening procedures include such sophisticated methodologies as immunoassays (inexpensive gauge of antibody response by drugs, used to screen large numbers of samples), gas chromatography, and mass spectrometry. (After a positive immunoassay is observed, gas chromatography with mass spectrometry is used—not only to confirm results, but also to identify the particular banned substance via its "molecular finger-print."]

Most athletic federations also now use "A" and "B" urine samples to eliminate potential problems such as chain of custody as well as clerical and/or tampering problems—all of which can produce a false positive. Essentially, the second sealed and untampered sample must corroborate the results of the "A" sample; if the two results don't jibe, the specimen is deemed negative.

As drug testing improves, athletes will assuredly become more knowledgeable in finding ways to beat the tests. And, of course, there will always be some rogue scientist or big company working on an even bigger, better, unable-to-be-detected drug.

Every player in the performance-enhancing drug field is aware of this truism: the chemists have been and always will be one step ahead of the dope detectives. It's like car thieves knowing about all the antitheft devices before they even hit the market; it's their job to know. And if they don't know something, you can be sure they'll soon find out.

This has certainly been the case with track and field athletes after 25 years of testing; working with their own trainers, physicians, and lab technicians, they've become adept at beating anything that the federations have thrown at them. Now, with random, more reliable testing in the NFL, football players are becoming increasingly savvy. It is a backhanded compliment to the drug policies of the current NFL régime that football players are now actively seeking knowledge from those experts in other sports who've effectively battled with the system for years.

Most sports federations and leagues now test athletes for recreational as well as performance-enhancing drugs. This is contrary to most drug tests in the workplace, which usually only screen for recreational drugs.

What then is the principle reason for drug testing? Is the

purpose to protect the health of the individual? Or is it to protect society? Is it to make the workplace safer? In sports, is it to return the athletic field to competitive balance? Or is it simply used to punish the "cheater"?

In my opinion, drug testing is definitely *not* used to protect the individual, at least in the sports world. I would maintain that the known risks are greater with an athlete's mere participation in sports such as boxing, hockey, and football (where there is a 100 percent injury rate) than with AAS use (the dangers of which are currently unknown).

As for making the workplace safer, no real attempt has been made to reduce the injury factor in those sports. In football, for example, we know that artificial turf increases the players' risk for certain injuries; yet there has been no attempt to eliminate these cheaper, easier-to-maintain surfaces from NFL stadiums.

Are we then protecting society from the increased size and aggression of AAS users? Again, in football, that's exactly what the fans pay to see: huge, fast, angry men colliding with vicious intensity.

Most sports organizations would argue that drug testing is done to return the athletic stadium/rink/ring/field/court/ arena to a more competitive balance. I would argue that it is a noble thought, but a most unrealistic goal. As long as athletic worth—compensated with immense fortune and fame—is measured by performance, athletes will do whatever they can to win, excel, and earn as much as they possibly can. There is too much money at stake to expect 20-year-old kids from poor backgrounds to use an ethical yardstick whenever they ponder a career move. As long as one athlete is using something to improve his or her performance, there will be at least one more athlete who wants to compete on the same level. And then another. And soon you have the same problem that we have now.

This simplistic philosophy inevitably creates two tiers of

athletes: the elite, well-connected few who have access to the state-of-the-art drugs and drug testing methods; and the honorable (or ignorant) masses who know they're competing at a distinct disadvantage (or who get caught). It doesn't take much for the member of the second tier to try and make the leap up.

It seems to me that when people talk about the "necessary evil" of drug testing, they're rarely the ones pissing in a cup. There's something very demeaning about having to void your bladder while some lab technician watches and waits. And how come, in most workplaces that screen for drugs, only the employees are tested?

I might not have felt so negatively about the process had Chuck Noll or Dan Rooney been standing in the adjoining stalls.

Some, of course, would argue that professional athletes are a breed apart. We should be held to a higher standard. We are, after all, Role Models.

Fair enough, I suppose, though some argue that an athlete owes his all to the public only when he's between the white lines. I'm not sure I agree, but I definitely do not believe that sports stars should be held to an unreasonably high standard either.

The sporting federations usually offer this argument when the ethics of drug testing are, well, tested. "We have to set an example for our kids," they contend.

Soon after Oklahoma's Brian Bosworth tested positive for steroids at the '87 Orange Bowl, the Seattle Seahawks of the NFL rewarded him with one of the largest contracts ever given a rookie linebacker. What message does that send to our kids? That you, too, can become rich and famous if you use performance-enhancing drugs? To impressionable young people, this is tacit, if not expressed, approval of steroid use.

Arnold Schwarzenegger, chairman of the President's

Council on Physical Fitness, is an admitted steroid user. I like Arnold's action movies as much as the next guy, but what kind of role model is that for kids?

In 1988, Florence Griffith-Joyner became one of the most visible female athletes in the world for her three gold medals (in the individual 100 and 200 meters and 4 x 100 relay) and one silver (4 x 400 relay) at the Seoul Olympics. She was presented as an attractive, intelligent woman who had achieved great success through hard work and a fierce determination. Yet most people in the track and field community—the ones who really *know*—claimed that she used steroids.

To argue the point, they compared photos, tapes, and records of Flo-Jo from 1984 to 1988; the physical differences were extraordinary. In 1988, she had all the classic symptoms of a woman using steroids—reduction of breast size, increased muscularity and masculine traits such as a deepened voice and facial hair (mustache). Her performance also improved 7 percent over her previous best, while Ben Johnson's "only" improved 4 percent.

She did a brilliant job of marketing herself, and of feminizing (some would say "disguising") her look with the exaggerated fingernails, the hair, the outfits, and tons of makeup. And she got out of the sport before undergoing further scrutiny.

Should Flo-Jo be considered a role model for starry-eyed young girls fighting for their piece of the American sports pie? It all depends on one's own moral compass (assuming she did indeed use steroids, and whether or not one feels that would be "cheating").

Ben Johnson was not the scandal of the 1988 Olympics. It was the way that the IOC and its apologists exploited Johnson's misfortune—moaning and whining about this "horrible" act as if it was truly aberrant behavior. Anita DeFrantz, an American member of the IOC, said after

Johnson's positive test: "To use drugs is cowardly, it's cheating, it's disgusting, it's vile."

That may all be true, but is she that misinformed or misguided as to believe that poor Ben Johnson was the only competitor in Seoul to have used a performance-enhancing drug? If these bureaucrats are so blind (or hypocritical), it's no wonder our drug policies are so ineffective.

It was also interesting how other prominent athletes joined in on the pummeling of Ben Johnson. Carl Lewis was particularly vocal and even vitriolic in his comments toward the man who originally beat him in the 100 meters. Lewis himself has been the subject of rumored AAS use. It's been speculated by reliable sources that Lewis tested positive for AAS in his "A" urine sample at the World Games at Helsinki in 1983, while—supposedly—the "B" sample was flushed by track and field officials in a cover-up that also affected some other "dirty" superstars.

I do acknowledge the danger of accusing people without concrete evidence. One could hide behind the "purported speculation" of "reliable sources" and advance any outlandish theory. And, admittedly, Carl is not the most well-liked athlete in the track and field community. But I do not offer these speculations lightly. As I mentioned, most athletes who take steroids—particularly in track and field—are very knowledgeable about their uses, including who is using. In this case, though, I would stress that there has been only rumor, no proof.

Dr. Charles Dubin, who headed the Ben Johnson inquiries in Toronto, reviewed 600 pages of testimony and then said he believed that most of the coaches and management involved in the Olympic world of athletics were involved in a "conspiracy of silence" when it came to the drug issue.

Bernd Heller, a West German sportscaster, disclosed during the Toronto hearings that 80 percent of the male track and field athletes who competed at Seoul in the 1988

Olympics had a "positive endocrine profile" (a new method of detecting AAS use that measures the altered output of pituitary hormones). Heller claimed he was told this by the head of the IOC's doping commission, Manfred Donike, a respected scientist who's developed much of the current drug testing metholology.

This conversation was reportedly off the record. With few exceptions, most of the major sports federations have chosen to play political football rather than publicly and openly acknowledge the enormity of the problem. They would apparently prefer to protect their asses (and equally fat assets) than take any real action.

I believe the only reason that the NFL, the IOC, and the other athletic establishments even have drug testing is to appease the public, as well as to relieve themselves of all legal, medical, and moral responsibilities.

Since the NFL had virtually no tests for steroids when I played, I didn't have to concern myself with beating them. My research during that time was mostly confined to finding the most effective drugs and learning how to prevent bodily damage or injury.

From other athletes, I discovered the simple technique of swimming. I'd heard about trainers who shot their racehorses with steroids, and then "swam" them in order to loosen the animals' connective tissue and joints and help their bodies adjust to the added muscular weight; apparently, this basis exercise worked as well with humans.

My first two six-week Dianabol cycles—as a sophomore in college and then again right before the pros—were supposedly supervised by physicians; but, in truth, the doctors gave me nothing but a prescription. Since the American Medical Association (AMA) had issued no guidelines for AAS dosages in athletes, I had to resort to trial and error.

As my teammates and I got more deeply involved in the drugs, we graduated from simple cycles of single steroids to stacks of greater dosages. I soon discovered that if I trained long and hard without drugs (this is called hitting the wall, or entering a catabolic state) and then went on cycle, my training would be appreciably more productive.

In 1984, I read my first book on the subject, Fred Hatfield's *Bodybuilding: A Scientific Approach*. A Ph.D., a former world-champion powerlifter, and well respected in the sports medicine community, Hatfield wrote about the most effective, safest ways of cycling the drugs, and I eventually tried his program of "descending doses." I met him when he was lecturing in the Pittsburgh area and asked about the best way to avoid muscle pulls. He told me to stay away from heavily androgenic drugs. Right then, I switched to a more anabolic-oriented program.

As I began to train for weightlifting competitions, I became even more knowledgeable and sophisticated in my cycling. I learned to expertly mix orals and injectables, and began using human chorionic gonadotropin (HCG) at the end of my cycles to help restimulate my natural testosterone production. I also discovered the benefits of antiestrogen drugs, which I took to alleviate or minimize the appearance of gynecomastia (male "breasts").

I never was a big fan of needles, but they became an integral part of my training regimen—like Ben-Gay or an Ace bandage. And let me tell you, it's not easy for a 300-pound man to give himself a shot in the rear. After a while, you figure out how to alternate sports—lower glute early in the week, upper glute later in the week—so as to avoid bruising (which is why most people "shoot the glute" and not the legs).

In four years of college and my first five years in the pros, I probably totalled 2,500 milligrams of steroids in four cycles. After that, my average weekly dose was probably about 400 milligrams. I know weightlifters who absorbed more than 2,500 milligrams in a *week*. (Therapeutic doses usually top out at 1,400 mg per week.) Ultimately, mega-doses can saturate receptor sites, thereby increasing health risks without any perceived performance benefits.

Hatfield's proposed one milligram of AAS per kilogram of body weight per day is probably the maximum "risk to benefit" dose one should consider. (I would strongly suggest that anyone using significant amounts of steroids, for whatever reasons, periodically take blood pressure checks, liver enzyme tests, and an electrocardiogram. And, of course, do it all under the supervision of a knowledgeable physician and maybe trainer.)

During a 15-year period of intermittent cycling, I used anabolic-androgenic steroids in 14 episodes (nine in the NFL), for less than 20 percent of my total training time (150 weeks over 15 years). Only once, over a three-week period, did I exceed 1,000 milligrams per week; and that was in 1985, around the time of my accelerated heart rate. I used 18 steroids at one time or another, though I never stacked more than five at a time.

I've been asked many times: If you had to do it all over again, would you use performance-enhancing drugs? Knowing what I now know, believing what I now believe, the answer would assuredly be: No, No, No.

But then again, if I had to do it all over again, I would not have been a professional football player.

11

POLITICAL
FOOTBALL
AND FALLOUT

THE NATIONAL FOOTBALL League—certainly during Pete Rozelle's 29-year reign as commissioner—basically tried to ignore the problem of steroids, hoping it would go away. There was plenty of breast-beating and image polishing, but no program with any real teeth in it. And very little heart.

Rozelle and the NFL were no doubt four-square against the use of steroids—they said so many times—but they didn't even start *announced* testing until 1987. This was two years after the *Sports Illustrated* article detailed extensive AAS usage in the NFL (in which Rozelle stated that "anabolic steroid use is not that big" in pro football), and, by most accounts, nearly 25 years since performance-enhancing drugs entered the league in San Diego.

Many NFL as well as high school and college coaches have encouraged their players to use performance-enhancing drugs. When any coach *suggests* that a player gain 20 pounds in the off-season, he might as well be writing out a prescription.

181

In 1983, two months after 19 athletes, including two Americans, tested positive at the Pan Am Games in Caracas, Venezuela, Rozelle sent a statement to all team coaches, physicians, trainers, and athletes that use of anabolic steroids "to achieve increased bulk, strength, stamina or similar physical and athletic attributes" would result in "appropriate disciplinary action (taken against) involved players or club personnel."

The language was intentionally vague. It never spelled out specific penalties. Suspensions? Fines? Expulsion? Nothing.

Rozelle's statement was posted in all locker rooms. And that was that—the extent of the NFL drug policy at that time.

In the fall of 1986, the NFL announced its plan to begin AAS testing during mini and training camps the following year. "Testing for steroids will be quite expensive," said Pete Rozelle, "but we intend to do it."

Around the same time, the NCAA began their own tests—also announced—before all bowl games. (The NCAA had proclaimed its drug testing plan nearly a year before it was implemented.)

Even with twelve months to prepare, 22 college players were dumb enough to test positive—including the brainy "Boz," Brian Bosworth. For all his overhyped shenanigans as a strutting, flamboyant, violent master of the game, the Oklahoma linebacker also promoted himself as a bright, articulate guy and a solid B student.

Well, maybe Oklahoma had some pretty lax academic standards back then, but I'd say that any player who gets caught in an announced test with a year to prepare ain't too bright.

What did the NFL do after the Boz tested positive for anabolic-androgenic steroids? It rewarded him with the then-largest contract ever given to a rookie linebacker.

What's the real message here, kids? That only a fool would say No. And that only a fool would believe the NFL was actually doing something to control the rampant us of anabolic-androgenic steroids by its players.

In 1987, 97 out of about 1,400 active NFL players (466 of whom were linemen) tested positive during training camp. A lot of bright guys in that class, too. That's 6 percent of the league in an *announced* test. A 1 percent yield in the Olympics is considered high, and yet most people acknowledge a serious steroid problem there.

What did Pete Rozelle and the NFL do to the players who tested positive for steroids in 1987? They sent around a little note to each one saying, in essence: "You tested positive."

In 1988, the NFL announced that any player who tested positive for steroids would be "subject to appropriate discipline by the commissioner."

The commissioner himself said: "Each instance in which a second positive test for (steroids) is confirmed will be handled on a case by case basis." In other words, they were going to pick and choose exactly who they wanted to punish and who would get off with a slap on the wrist.

In March 1989, at the owners' meeting in Palm Springs, Rozelle announced his plan to step down as commissioner as soon as a suitable replacement could be found. In addition, Rozelle revealed that any player caught using steroids would be suspended for "a minimum of 30 days from the time you are advised of the test results, or until your system is shown to be clear of steroids and/or masking agents, whichever is *later*."

This later proclamation came five months *before* the actual drug test. When confronted with the loss of a paycheck, the numbers went from 97 to 13 (about 1 percent of all players). This didn't mean, of course, that there were necessarily fewer players using—only fewer players using during the testing period.

Rozelle and Dr. Forest Tennant, the NFL's drug advisor, both made statements to the effect that "six percent" or "one percent" was just a tiny portion of the pro football population; and, they contended, while there may have been a few more guys out there beating the system, it was a neglible amount.

In essence, they ignored the compelling argument that a player would have to be pretty damn stupid to get caught in an announced test; and that if *only* 13 players got caught, then the actual number of users was likely much, much greater. It's ludicrous how an entity as large and powerful as the NFL could successfully hide itself like an ostrich from the realities of the real world—and from the consequences of their nonactions.

No doubt some players did stay away from steroids once they saw that the NFL was finally serious. But many others—by becoming more knowledgeable about human growth hormone and testosterone manipulating—merely learned how to circumvent the tests. They discovered how with certain steroids, they could stay on their cycles during the off-season up until one month before the season began and still test clean.

In 1990, under new commissioner Paul Tagliabue, the NFL began random testing for steroids. Interestingly, this pronouncement was revealed during Super Bowl week, on the heels of Washington, D.C. TV station WJLA's allegation that Tennant had covered up the results of a positive test for cocaine by three white quarterbacks.

The allegations seriously threatened the credibility of the NFL's program, and of Dr. Tennant. Desperately needing a P.R. victory, Tagliabue announced the random tests to take off some of the heat and to show how responsible the league was becoming in dealing with the drug problem.

Once more, the league's actions seemed driven more by a concern for public image than for its players. (Moreover, the NFL's random system remains flawed. Players who've previously tested positive for steroids are sampled as often, or not, as those who have never taken the drugs. Also, the NFL still refuses to use an independant testing facility.)

The story of the three quarterbacks—though many people believed it to be true—was never confirmed. As a result of this incident, and several other purported "indiscretions" which later surfaced, Tennant soon left his position as NFL drug czar to pursue other interests.

With all due respect, Dr. Tennant had no business being offered the job in the first place. His main credential was that he had run a slew of methadone clinics in California. He apparently knew very little about steroids. (After he got the job, he immediately called Dr. Bob Goldman of the Chicago College of Ostepathic Medicine, a knowledgeable man in the field, to pick his brain about AAS use.) Unfortunately, that didn't prevent Dr. Tennant from making statements that were medically and scientifically false. Such as: steroids do not help in the recuperation of injuries. And: sterility is a side effect of anabolic steroids.

In its July 10, 1989, issue, *Sports Illustrated* published a detailed report by Richard Demak and Jerry Kirshenbaum entitled "The NFL Fails Its Drug Test."

"[Rozelle] has ruled over the NFL's program like Jehovah, sitting as judge, jury and prosecutor of drug cases," the authors contended. "However, nothing Rozelle has done opens him to second-guessing more than his appointment of Dr. Forest Tennant Jr. as the league's drug advisor. . . . In carrying out his NFL duties, [Tennant's] administrative competence and adherence to accepted drug-testing standards have been found seriously wanting."

How so?

According to Demak and Kirshenbaum: "League officials

have misstated the dimensions of drug use among players, exaggerating or underestimating it, depending on the public relations needs of the moment. They have seldom bothered to distinguish between players who are addicted and those who have used drugs recreationally. And they have misappropriated drug testing, using a medical tool for punitive purposes."

In 1990, Dr. John Lombardo was named the new NFL advisor for anabolic steroids and performance-enhancing drugs. As the medical director of the sports medicine section at the Cleveland Clinic Foundation, Dr. Lombardo was much better versed on steroids than his predecessor. In 1989 he cowrote the paper "Anabolics in Athletes" with Dr. Jim Wright, director of Sports Science Consultants of Indiannapolis, and my friend, Penn State professor Dr. Chuck Yesalis). Whether or not he will get to put any of his expertise to practice, however, is yet to be determined.

When Lyle Alzado went public with his belief that performance-enhancing drugs caused his brain cancer, also disclosing that he took substantial doses of steroids throughout his 14-year NFL career, and even beat a league drug test in 1990 during his unsuccessful comeback, Dr. Lombardo was conspicuously silent. It was not necessarily by choice.

In fact, the New York Times reported that Greg Aiello, the NFL's director of communications, said that "the NFL's current drug advisor, Dr. John Lombardo of Ohio State University, would not be allowed to comment on the league's steroid policy and testing procedures." Instead, it was left to Mr. Aiello, the league flack, to offer his studied opinion.

"There's no question that steroids is a dangerous business," Aiello said. "That's a message that we've delivered to our players for many years. Steroids is a banned substance in the NFL and we have continued to strengthen our steroids-abuse program over the years."

In the same *Times* account, our old friend Dr. Forest Tennant took a little bite out of the hand that used to feed him.

"There was no discouragement of the use of the steroids by team doctors prior to 1986," Tennant said. "As I made my first rounds, it was apparent that steroids was a great problem. It was also very clear that we had ignorance of them and [had condoned] them in a certain sense."

Contrary to the proclamations made during his league tenure, Tennant contended "that you had half the linemen and linebackers using [steroids] in 1986. Now, I'd say that it's down to 20–25 percent."

Tennant also expressed criticism of the NFL's current drug policy. "Random testing only tests a handful of people, and it doesn't get to the guys who are known to have used them."

It's interesting to note how Dr. Tennant had gotten his mind right in just the year or so since he left his NFL post. Yet he exposed a still-profound lack of AAS expertise in commenting on Lyle Alzado's situation.

"With the levels of anabolic steroids that some of these guys are taking, I do not see how some of these fellows will not develop cancer," Tennant said. "Alzado is not the first steroids user to develop cancer. He's just the first famous person. He's a signal. He's going to be the first in a long line of these people with cancer."

Again, the facts contradict the doctor's opinions. There have been three documented cancer (liver, kidney, and prostate) fatalities stemming from AAS use. And there have been no other cases connecting steroids to T-cell lymphoma, Alzado's rare brain cancer.

Tennant's know-nothing yet inflammatory comment was typical of the "reefer madness" mentality that overtook much of the media and the public in response to Lyle's cancer and admitted steroid use. The real experts were more circumspect.

"There is zero correlation between brain tumors and steroids," said Dr. Gary Wadler of the Cornell University Medical College, a noted authority on drugs in sports. The news coverage of the Alzado story, he maintained, was based on a false premise that in turn led to "a media feeding frenzy [that] wasn't responsible.

"I've talked to everyone and his brother in the field, scientists, endocrinologists," Wadler continued, "and no one sees any evidence of relationship between his story and his cancer."

Lyle's own physician admitted his own—as well as the medical community's—ignorance on the matter. "No one knows if growth hormones or anabolic steroids cased Lyle's cancer," said Dr. Robert Huizenga, an internist who was also the Raiders' team doctor in the early eighties. "There is no evidence. This is Lyle's theory that it caused cancer. I'm not disputing that. But there is no scientific evidence that anabolic steroids or growth hormone caused the rare brain cancer that Lyle has."

Huizenga said he first warned Lyle of the possibly damaging side effects of steroids as early as 1982, but that Lyle obviously chose to make his own decisions.

"I was wild about winning," Lyle said in the July 8, 1991, issue of *Sports Illustrated*, giving that as one of the reasons for his AAS use. (On the magazine's cover, the headline "I LIED," was bannered across Lyle's face—disease-ravaged, but still wild-eyed—along with: FORMER NFL STAR LYLE ALZADO NOW ADMITS TO MASSIVE USE OF STEROIDS AND HUMAN GROWTH HORMONE—AND BELIEVES THEY CAUSED HIS INOPERABLE BRAIN CANCER.

In the first-person account, told to writer Shelley Smith, Lyle said that he first took steroids in order to play college football at Yankton College in South Dakota because "I had the speed but not the size." The first steroid he used was Dianabol, about 50 milligrams a day.

"I remember a couple of weeks later someone mentioned how my biceps seemed to look bigger," he said. "I was so proud. I was lifting weights so much that the results were pretty immediate and dramatic. I went from 190 pounds to 220 by eating a lot, and then I went up to 300 pounds from the steroids. People say that steroids can make you mean and moody, and my mood swings are incredible. That's what made me a football player, my moods on the field."

Remind you of anyone?

Lyle and I have much in common. He has T-cell lymphoma, a rare form of brain cancer. I have dilated cardiomyopathy, a relatively uncommon heart disease. Both of us have admitted significant AAS use during our pro football careers. We both believe that a large percentage of NFL players have used or are still using performance-enhancing drugs. And we both strongly agree that AAS use by kids should be stopped, and extensive research begun.

One of the areas in which we differ is his belief that steroids caused his illness. I am not convinced that his disease or mine were necessarily caused by the use of AAS. To date, Lyle's is the only known case of brain cancer—while mine is the single reported instance of dilated cardiomyopathy—in more than one (and possibly as high as three) million AAS users.

I should note, however, that Lyle cites his use of human growth hormone (HGH) as the cause of his illness, while I never used HGH. I also believe that *megadoses* of certain performance-enhancing drugs (including steroids and HGH) can suppress the immune system and create an opening for any number of life-threatening conditions.

Several physicians have expressed a similar opinion, but there hasn't been much, if any, scientific corroboration. I have nothing more to go on than an accelerated heart rate after my megadosage in 1985, but I feel in my mind (and gut) that this is a distinct probability.

There are, of course, other factors that could have contributed to both of our rare conditions: environment, recreational drug use, stress, and genetic predisposition. Again, in the case of my cardiomyopathy, alcohol abuse has been cited as a possible link.

Lyle and I differed greatly in the amount of steroids taken and the length of the specific cycles. I cycled 14 times sprinkled over a 15-year period, only once (in '85) exceeding 1,000 milligrams per week.

"I started taking anabolic steroids in 1969, and I never stopped," Lyle said. "Not when I retired from the NFL in 1985. Not ever . . .

"I'm convinced that my biggest mistake was never going off cycle," he continued. "According to the guys around the gym, if you go on steroids for six to eight weeks, then you're supposed to stop for the same number of weeks. Me, I'd be on the stuff for 10 or 12 weeks, and then I'd go off for only two, maybe three weeks, and I'd feel that was enough. It was addicting, mentally addicting."

I can't imagine that—never going off cycle, always pumped and primed and ready to snap.

"I became very violent on the field," Lyle said. "Off it, too. I did things only crazy people do. Once in 1979 in Denver a guy sideswiped my car, and I chased him up and down hills through the neighborhoods. I did that a lot. I'd chase a guy, pull him out of his car, beat the hell out of him."

Lyle got away with his actions because he was a professional football player. A Brown. A Bronco. A Raider. Civilian casualties were acceptable during the week, as long as you kicked some big-time NFL butt on Sundays. Then all was forgiven.

Our society seems unwilling or unable to deal with *its* own addiction to football, and to sports in general. We say we're against these drugs, yet we're out there every Sunday screaming for 300-pound linemen to "rip their lungs out!" We want to ooh and ah at the extraordinary feats these athletes perform, yet we don't really want to know how they got this way—usually concocted in some laboratory. And we don't want to acknowledge the price that is being paid by the athletes to amaze and entertain us.

We can't just keep blaming the so-called institutional powers. It's too easy to criticize individuals such as Chuck Noll, Pete Rozelle, and Forest Tennant for their part in the continuing AAS problem. It's time that the man on the street, or the woman in the stands, took some responsibility as well.

After I heard about Lyle's health predicament and the price he was paying, I felt as numb and depressed as when I learned about former NFL defensive lineman John Matuszak's death at 38 of a reported heart attack. I remember both of them as young, strong, wild, and worthy opponents on the football field. Their premature plight was also a sobering reminder of my own mortality.

I was again reminded of the similarities between Lyle's situation and mine. While I was not merely as famous, flamboyant, or perhaps as deathly ill, I could relate to much of what he and his family were going through: the debilitating fight against a rare disease; the first-person account in *Sports Illustrated*; the public admission of personal AAS use, along with the claims of widespread use in the NFL; the subsequent denial (or silence) by the league. It even struck me that we both wore the number 77 during our playing days.

There was one more touch of irony: When I revealed the extent of my steroid usage in *Sports Illustrated* in 1985, the writer of the piece, Jill Lieber, told me that she had been speaking to one other active player. He was, she said, very open in detailing his current AAS use, but very adamant about not wanting to go public. He would provide background as long as she didn't provide his name.

That player was, of course, Lyle Alzado.

On the heels of Lyle's disclosures, another steroid-related story affected me personally and deeply.

On July 24, 1991, late in the afternoon, I received a call from a woman I had never met. "You don't know me," she said, "but I'm Terry Long's girlfriend." Terry was an acquaintance, a veteran Steeler offensive lineman to whom I had recently mailed some AAS-related material.

"I don't know who else to call," she said. "I got your name from some papers on Terry's desk." The woman sounded distraught, and I asked her what was wrong.

"Terry's upstairs," she said. "I think he's just swallowed some rat poison, and doesn't want me to call the paramedics."

What!?!

"He said he'll just try it again," she said. "He recently found out that he'd tested positive for steroids. He thinks his career is over. He told me his life is over."

I couldn't believe what I was hearing. I was trying to stay calm, so she would stay calm. Good thing she couldn't hear me shaking.

"You did the right thing calling the ambulance," I told her. "He'll thank you for it later.

"Oh, and whatever you do," I cautioned, "don't let the media get hold of this."

Any good reporter has sources in hospitals and precinct houses—people who are often paid for their information. It took all of a day before the story was splashed all over the tabloids and the television; they were reporting that, prior to ingesting the poison, Terry had "started a car in a closed garage at his home" before his girlfriend "found him and called for help." The story was covered nationally, but in Pittsburgh it was big news.

The front page headline of the July 26th *Pittsburgh Post-Gazette* read: STEELER SWALLOWS POISON . . . GUARD TERRY LONG HOSPITALIZED; HAD FAILED TEAM'S STEROID TEST.

My phone began ringing nonstop. Somehow the media had found out that I had spoken to Terry's girlfriend. The reporters asked if I had talked to Terry.

I lied. I said that I hadn't.

The truth is, I spoke to Terry Long at home before he was admitted to Allegheny General, the same hospital in which I had spent some recovery time. I told Terry that what he had tested positive for—the high testosterone ratio—was appealable; several Olympic athletes had gotten their rulings reversed.

I tried to cheer him up with any number of platitudes: Everything'll be fine. Your career is not over. You can win your appeal.

Terry was basically inconsolable. He couldn't see a life beyond football. "If you don't believe me," I said, "Please call Chuck Yesalis."

Fortunately, Terry did call Chuck and was persuaded to finally go to the hospital. For my part I regret lying to the press, but I was trying to protect a man's life. Terry's psyche was too fragile; I didn't want to stir up any feelings that could affect him negatively. The only quotes I gave to the papers involved the steroid tests themselves.

Back in February, after the Steelers had failed to place him on their B protected list, 32-year-old Terry Long said: "It's a bad feeling. It leaves you hollow. I thought I had maybe a couple of years left in me. You have to face it—I'm getting old. I'm not doing some of the things they want me to do.

"Only the fortunate ones get to leave when they want to. I probably won't get to leave when I want to."

Terry Long didn't want to leave. Neither did Lyle Alzado. Nor did I. Few of us get to leave when we want to. Few of us are able to seamlessly begin new lives after football. Few of us can initially see that there is life beyond football.

Many of the stories focusing on Terry Long and Lyle Alzado have romanticized the tragic glory of the doomed gladiator: the noble savage giving up his body, and ultimately his life.

But to what end?

That's the tragedy. There's no glory in dying for a *sport*.

12

PRESENT
AND FUTURE

AS A YOUNG boy, I bought into the myth of football. I was taught early on that the game was simulated war, and you did what you had to do to win. I was not alone.

"It's all I cared about," Lyle Alzado said, "winning, winning. All I thought about. I never talked about anything else."

Coaches didn't talk about much else. It was, they dutifully echoed Vince Lombardi's line, the only thing.

I fully accepted this mandate. And I gloried in it. I played on a winning team in high school and college, and then I was drafted onto one of the most successful teams in pro football history. I did my small part—whatever it took to get the job done.

I learned a lot about myself. More than most "games," football reveals much about character. You soon find out who responds well to pressure, and who will fold in the clutch; you discover who's in it for the challenge or the fun, and who'd just as soon sell out his mother for a dime.

195

I regret few things in my life, but I do regret selling myself out to the system by using drugs to compete. I regret being so overwhelmed by the game that I became a creature of it.

As I became more caught up in it, I learned how the system derived its power—from young, naïve men who wholeheartedly believed in it, and who would do anything their leaders told them to in order to triumph.

Ultimately I learned that one *can* just say no.

If, at age 10 or 12, my son (or daughter) comes to me—as I did to my parents—begging to play pee-wee football, I will gently tell the child: "No."

I don't believe that little kids should be outfitted in body armor and sent out to butt heads, certainly not while they're still growing (a fracture through the growth plate at this age could cause leg-length discrepancy and angular deformities).

There's altogether too much emphasis on winning in kids' sports, and I'd suggest that we eliminate competitive games up to the age of twelve or thirteen. The goal should be exercise and education—expending the effort while learning new skills. Success should not be determined by standings; it should be gauged by enjoyment. Fun is the only true measure at that age. There's time enough to become mercenaries.

If President Bush had tapped me, instead of Arnold Schwarzenegger as chairman of his physical fitness program, I would stress intramural sports at all levels, with a focus on learning lifetime fitness skills. On the high school level, I'd suggest that we eliminate TV coverage of events; eliminate state championships; reduce the length of the season as well as the number and intensity of practices; and increase rewards and recognition for academic achievement.

For college students, I'd work toward eliminating athletic scholarships, basing them instead on need. I'd institute frequent unscheduled, nonpunitive drug tests throughout the calendar year; direct all university donations to the general fund, not the athletic department; require equal sharing of TV and bowl receipts, try and take the pressure off coaches and players to win at all costs; and establish tenure tracks for coaches. In fact, we should use the same criteria for coaches as we use for other teachers: how they rank as educators, how they interact with kids, and so forth.

Right now, health permitting, my goal is to be a history teacher, probably on the college level. (After I go back for my undergraduate degree, I intend to go to grad school—maybe even get a doctorate.) But under the right circumstances—the right administration (and administrator)—I'd love to teach high school history and coach high school football.

I would try to do things a little differently than most coaches: We'd practice in pads only once a week; we'd emphasize technique, with chalkboard sessions and walk-through drills (both of which would prevent getting needlessly whacked around in practice); and, most importantly, we'd try to have fun.

I'd also try to build camaraderie with my high school charges—not only to win football games, but, more importantly (and though I promise to keep my coach's cliché output to a minimum), to build character.

There's no place in coaching for negativism and fear. Kids should hear how well they're doing, not how they're constantly screwing up. I'd compliment these kids as often as I could.

I'd tell them: "If I have to yell at you, that means I don't belong here." I'd also promise: "I won't ever embarrass you. I'm just going to teach you how to play." And: "We're definitely going to have some fun . . . and who knows? We may even win a few games."

The best thing about this speech is that I just gave it—at

summer orientation for the Trinity High School football team. After my friend and former teammate Ted Petersen got the job as head coach at Trinity, in Washington, Pennsylvania, he asked me to coach the offensive line. "If you're up to it physically, Steve," Ted said, "I'd love to have you work with me."

I checked with my doctor. She said that as long as I didn't exert myself too much, it shouldn't be a problem. She also said that I could begin light workouts on my own.

So in preparation for high school football season this fall, and in order to tone some of these muscles that have atrophied over the past three years, I've begun an easy regimen: working out at least four days a week for no more than an hour at a time; no straining; very deliberate repetitions. The majority of the exercises are with 50 to 60 pounds—in the old days, I'd warm up with twice that—with maybe a whopping 135 pounds on the bench press. It feels great to work out again, and very gratifying to be able to implement some of my theories with these kids.

The experimental drugs I've been taking for the cardiomyopathy seem to be working, and the doctor says my condition has stabilized "for the time being." I'm as fulfilled and optimistic as I've ever been in my life.

Of course, the reality is, I still need a heart transplant. My weight is up to 304, which my doctor says is too much for me to carry. Because of all the drugs I took in the past, my body chemistry is different. My body is different. Because my muscle memory is still there, I'll always be bigger. It doesn't matter if I eat a lot or not, my physique has been permanently altered.

One of the prime motivating forces in my life as I strive to get well is to be fit enough to travel. I learned relatively late in life that there's an entire world beyond the hashmarks, and I want to see it all.

I want to see the pyramids. I want to see the Western

Wall of Solomon's Temple and the well-preserved temple at Angkor Wat. I want to see the ruins of Greece, Babylon, and Mesopotamia. I'm teaching myself Russian, German, Spanish, and French so I can communicate with the people I meet and learn more about their culture and their way of life. Then I can come back and teach my students all the facets of history, present and past.

I suppose there's a very real possibility that I won't ever marry. But if I meet a woman along the way who shares my interests and who wants to be part of them, that'll be terrific. Kids of my own? We'll just have to wait and see on that, too.

I'm thirty-six years old. It's taken me about half of most men's lifetime to find out who I am, and I'd like a fair shot at discovering who I will become.

For a long time, I was simply Steve Courson, football player. Fans, coaches, and even some of my teammates could only see me as that (perhaps they defined themselves this way). Yet I always felt that it was such a limiting description.

The normal career expectancy of an NFL player is four years; I stayed more than twice that. When I first got sick, the doctors said my life expectancy was likely three to five years. I've made it through three, and I'm hoping to stick around a lot longer.

I'd be lying if I said I didn't think about death. But I don't dwell on it. It just makes me want to do as much as I can in whatever time I have left. And it definitely puts things in stark perspective. I don't get angry at the piddly stuff anymore. I don't have the time or patience for wasted anger.

I never was a material guy. Even when I was making $300,000 and could afford a Mercedes, I preferred to drive a camouflage Blazer. I lived in a small townhouse when I could have afforded a suburban mansion. I had the money, and I had the glory. But I knew then it was hollow, and now I truly don't miss any of it.

My ultimate dream is to buy a piece of land in Montana, near enough to a school so I could teach and coach—a place where I can build a cabin, raise some horses and dogs (Labrador retrievers), and grow vegetables in a garden. In forty or fifty years or so, when I'm old and fat and tired, I'd like to die working in my garden. In the meantime, I'd invite my buddies out to hunt and fish. And every July 4th I'd throw a big bash for my closest friends. We'd eat from a pig on a spit, dance to a country and western band, and laugh until we drop.

Right now, it's only a dream about a place I've yet to visit, about a day I may never see.

A great songwriter once sang something about those dreams only "in your head."

They're in my heart, too.

APPENDIX

AFTER I TESTIFIED before the Biden hearings in May 1989, I received a call from another committee witness, Dr. Charles Yesalis, a professor from Penn State. He said that I had done my homework.

We soon became friends. I read a copy of the survey that he had done of high school students and wondered whether we could do the same thing with pro football players. We talked to Bill Fralic and then to Doug Allen and Mike Kenn of the NFL Players Association.

"It's the best [survey] I've ever seen," Kenn, NFLPA president, told *The National*. "The only problem with the survey is that it's six or seven pages long. And I've never seen a player who will look at anything more than a couple of pages."

The NFLPA endorsed it and even kicked in some mailing costs. Penn State donated some computer time to the project, and I put in about $1,700 of my own money.

With input from the NFLPA, Chuck Yesalis and I formulated what ultimately became a 10-page questionnaire—60 multiple-choice questions in all.

Players were asked if they had used steroids or human growth hormone; where and how they got them; whether they trusted the validity or fairness of the NFL's drug testing program; and what was the primary influence on their use of these drugs. The method we used is known as systemic survey research, and essentially consists of using self-reported anonymous results.

The NFLPA mailed the surveys out in the summer of 1990 to the home addresses of approximately 1,600 NFL players on 28 teams. Unfortunately, only 120 players (7.5 percent of the NFL) returned the questionnaire to the NFLPA headquarters in Washington, D.C. They were then sent to Dr. Yesalis for analysis. Of the 120 players who responded, just over half were down linemen.

The poor response rate is obviously a critical aspect of the study. We cannot make any final assessments based on this low return. But we can get a sense of the view from within.

In the *Sports Illustrated* article on Lyle Alzado, his doctor, Robert Huizenga, was asked: "Why don't we know more about steroid usage by athletes and its effects?"

Huizenga said: "There are very few studies, and, frankly, the best group that could be studied and give useful information is NFL players. We—all the doctors of the clubs—agreed to back a study. We have not been embraced by the players' union or the league."

I don't know when Dr. Huizenga tried to pitch his study, probably before ours. It's indeed unfortunate, though, that even with the sanction of their association, most NFL players are reluctant to admit or discuss their AAS usage. (This past spring I proposed to a group of retired NFL players that we initiate a confidential, long-term study to follow the players' future health histories, comparing steroid users with non-users. The players indicated that they would comply with such a study.)

It is interesting to note that of the survey respondents who were asked to estimate the use of steroids among their fellow players, the percentages were quite close to the participants' self-reported levels (32 percent of the league vs. 28 percent of own use).

Also of interest: After the Alzado furor, the NFL finally acknowledged that approximately 30 percent of its players have

used steroids. Prior to this admission, its spokesmen were cling-
ing to those feeble "1" or "6" percent estimates.

The NFL is slowly coming to grips with the fact that it has a
problem, but it still seems to be everyone else's problem. Virginia
Cowart, a medical writer and co-author (with Jim Wright) of
Anabolic Steroids—Altered States, interviewed about half of the
NFL's team doctors.

"All the physicians admitted that 'there definitely is a steroid
problem' in the league, " she said, "But they all indicated that it
was on the 'other teams.'" None apparently wanted to take
responsibility for what was going on in his own backyard. And all
the drug tests in the world won't change that attitude.

Again, due to the low response rate, we can't generalize the
level of AAS use in the NFL beyond our sample (we still believe
the percentage to be appreciably higher). The findings do, however, make a very compelling argument that further research
must be done. The subsequent questions raised by both the Lyle
Alzado and Terry Long stories strongly emphasize this point.

Until the athletes themselves come forward in great numbers,
these surveys will be, at best, educated guesses.

ANABOLIC STEROID USE AMONG SELF-SELECTED SAMPLE OF NFL PLAYERS

Charles E. Yesalis, Sc.D.*
Stephen P. Courson

ABSTRACT

For several decades the level of anabolic steroid use in the National Football League (NFL) has been the subject of controversy. Estimates of the incidence of use, however, have been based on either anecdotal accounts or the results of drug tests, both of which have significant shortcomings. In 1990, with the support of the NFL Players Association, we attempted to survey more than 1,600 NFL players regarding their attitudes and behavior related to steroid use; unfortunately, only 120 players (7.5%) elected to participate in the study. Twenty-eight percent of all respondents and 67 percent of offensive lineman reported that they had used steroids at some time in their lives. However, only 3 percent of the participants acknowledged use in the past twelve months. Steroid use was generally initiated in college, with none of the users reporting use during high school. Half of the players

*Professor, Health Policy and Administration and Exercise and Sport Science, Pennsylvania State University. 115 Henderson Building, University Park, PA 16802. © 1991 by Charles E. Yesalis and Stephen P. Courson. Reprinted by permission.

thought anabolic steroid use had decreased over the past four years, and 87 percent believed that the random testing program initiated in 1990 would further decrease use. The majority of respondents, however, did not trust the accuracy or fairness of the testing program in place during the 1989 season. While the large majority of players want steroid use curtailed, they believe that the NFL primarily views steroid use as a public relations problem and that the coaches are, at best, indifferent to the players' use of these drugs. Because of the low response rate in this study, the data and the conclusions offered must be regarded with caution in relation to the totality of NFL players.

Anabolic steroid use in sports has been the subject of controversy for several decades. Part of the controversy involves a disagreement over the level of steroid use among players in the National Football League (NFL). Rumors and anecdotes as well as testimonials by current and former NFL players going back to the 1960s[1] have resulted in estimates of drug use as high as 90 percent[2–5]. On the other hand, the NFL management disagrees that the problem is widespread and cites the results of their drug testing program, which found 6 percent of players to be users in 1987 and less than 1 percent in both 1989 and 1990.

However, the results of drug testing, particularly announced tests, are often inaccurate indicators of the prevalence of steroid use[6–7]. In particular, the specificity of drug tests for some anabolic steroids, especially the oral agents and the esters of testosterone, is thought to be poor[6–9].

Yet another means of assessing the level of anabolic steroid use among athletes is by systematic survey research employing anonymous, self-report questionnaires. This method has been used among high school and college athletes[10–12] and yields steroid use rates significantly greater than those obtained from drug tests[6]. However, it is believed that even the results of self-report surveys still underestimate the true level of drug use, particularly among élite athletes[13].

To our knowledge, no systematic survey of anabolic steroid use in the NFL has been reported in the literature. In the spring of 1990, we conducted such a survey with the approval and support of the NFL Players Association (NFLPA).

METHODS

The NFLPA mailed a survey instrument containing sixty multiple-choice questions, along with a stamped, self-addressed envelope, to the homes of approximately 1,600 active NFL players on 28 teams. The NFLPA actively participated in the development of the questionnaire, and a letter explaining the purpose of the survey as well as its anonymous (i.e., regarding the identity
of the individual and team) and confidential nature was cosigned by the president of the NFLPA and the chair of the NFLPA's Health and Safety Committee. This study was approved by the Pennsylvania State University's Office for the Protection of Human Subjects.

In addition to measuring the incidence of steroid use, the survey assessed the attitudes and opinions of participants related to the efficacy, accuracy, and fairness of the NFL drug testing program as well as the players' perceptions of the NFL's motives for drug testing. Signs and symptoms of steroid use were identified among those who reported using the drug.

RESULTS

Only 120 of the 1,600 potential respondents (≈7.5%) returned the questionnaire, 65 percent of whom had played in the NFL for more than five years. The low response rate is a critical aspect of the study and impacts the extent to which the findings can be generalized to all NFL players (see Discussion).

When the participants were asked what percentage of their fellow NFL players they believed had *ever* used anabolic steroids, the mean response was 32 percent; the estimate of use among fellow players for the *past 12 months* was 19 percent. When respondents were asked, "Have you *ever* used anabolic steroids to assist your training in high school, in college or in the NFL?" 28 percent answered yes; of offensive linemen, 67 percent responded yes. However, only 3 percent of all respondents admitted using steroids during the past twelve months. Of those who acknowledged prior steroid use, none used the drugs in high school, while 25 percent used them only in college, 31 percent used them only in the NFL, and 44 percent used the drugs both in college and the NFL.

The approximate number of steroid cycles reported by the participants is shown in Table 1, with the median response category being 2–5 cycles.

Table 1

Approximate Number of Anabolic Steroid Cycles
Taken during Lifetime

# of cycles	% of respondents
1	18.1%
2–5	36.4%
6–10	36.4%
11–15	6.1%
greater than 15	3.0%

All respondents were asked to assess whether or not the level of steroid use had changed during the "past four years." Thirty-nine percent believed that the level of use had remained the same or increased, whereas 50 percent believed that use had decreased (11 percent answered "don't know"). Among steroid users, 41 percent thought use had increased or stayed the same and 56 percent felt use had decreased.

Of the study participants who acknowledged steroid use, a number reported signs and symptoms commonly associated with such use (Table 2). Users reported an average of 6.3 signs or symptoms, while 78 percent of users reported 3 or more signs or symptoms. It is interesting to note that with the exception of increased aggression, sex drive, appetite, and fluid retention, no one sign or symptom is experienced by the majority of steroid users.

When asked if they would "like to see the use of anabolic steroids in the NFL stopped," 87 percent of all survey participants (Table 3) and 79 percent of steroid users responded "definitely yes." Similarly, 78 percent of the steroid users stated that they

Table 2

Self-Reported Signs and Symptoms
While Taking Anabolic Steroids

Signs/Symptoms	%of Respondents		
	Yes	No	Don't Know
acne	29%	65%	6%
greasy skin or hair	21	73	6
scalp hair loss	15	79	6
increased body hair	27	58	15
increased number of headaches	12	76	12
nosebleeds	3	91	6
yellowing of skin or eyes	9	88	3
increased irritability or aggression	65	29	6
depression	23	73	3
difficulty sleeping	32	62	6
euphoria	30	61	9
increased sex drive	70	24	6
decreased sex drive	15	79	6
gynecomastia	12	82	6
fluid retention	68	26	6
frequent urge to urinate	15	73	12
muscle spasms	9	85	6
enlarged prostate	3	71	26
altered liver enzymes	6	68	26
altered cholesterol levels	15	61	24
elevated blood pressure	35	53	12
increased appetite	62	32	6
decreased appetite	3	87	10

would stop using steroids if they "were *absolutely* convinced" that their competitors did not use them. Moreover, at least 80 percent of steroid users expressed the intention of "definitely" stopping steroid use if it was proven *beyond doubt* that they would lead to sterility, impotence, or increased risk of liver cancer or a heart attack (Table 3).

When queried about their perceptions of the NFL management's attitudes on the issue of steroid use, 60 percent of the players in this study felt that their coaches either approved or did not care about anabolic steroid use; only 27 percent believed that NFL coaches disapproved of use. However, 76 percent of anabolic steroid users in this sample stated that their coaches approved or did not care and only 12 percent felt that their coaches somewhat disapproved of their use; none of the users believed that their

Table 3

Attitudes Regarding Anabolic Steroid Use

Question: Definitely	Definitely Yes	Probably Yes	Not Sure	Probably No	No
Would like to see the use of anabolic steroids in the NFL stopped	87%	5%	5%	2%	1%
Would stop using anabolic steroids if *absolutely* convinced competitors no longer used them	78	18	4	—	—
Would discontinue use of anabolic steroids if *proven* beyond doubt they would:					
· lead to permanent sterility	80	13	3	3	—
· double your risk of liver cancer	90	6	3	—	—
· triple risk of heart attack before age 50	90	10	—	—	—
· lead to impotence	81	19	—	—	—

coaches strongly disapproved. In addition, 78 percent of all respondents believed that concern over "its public image," as opposed to concerns of health or fair play, was the *principal reason* why the NFL established drug testing.

In assessing the efficacy of the NFL drug testing program in place during 1989,[†] 43 percent of players (47 percent of users)

†The 1989 drug testing program consisted of an announced test in preseason training camp. In 1990 the NFL initiated a random testing program where players were subjected to year-round drug screening.

somewhat or strongly disagreed that the program significantly reduced the use of steroids, versus 45 percent who agreed (44 percent of users). Approximately half of the participants in the study expressed a lack of trust in the accuracy and the fairness of the NFL program in place in 1989 (Table 4); the level of mistrust among steroid users was only slightly higher. On the other hand, 87 percent of all respondents and 94 percent of steroid users believed that a frequent (up to four times a year) random testing program (similar to the one instituted in 1990) would "somewhat or dramatically decrease" steroid use.

Table 4
Attitudes on Drug Testing

Definitely:	Definitely	Probably	Not	Probably	
	Yes	Yes	Sure	No	No
Trust the *accuracy* of the NFL drug testing program	6%	33%	11%	25%	25%
Trust the *fairness* of the NFL drug testing program	13	25	13	25	24

DISCUSSION

This paper presents information on anabolic steroid use among a small sample of a heretofore unstudied population, NFL players. This population is important in that it represents the highest level of competition in one of the most popular sports in our country, with over one million participants at the high school level. Moreover, football, because of its strength and power requirements, lends itself to the use of anabolic steroids.

The critical limitation of this current study is the markedly low rate of participation (≈7.5%). Given this low response rate, are the findings presented here important? We believe they are in that they represent the views of a group of insiders in what was previously a "closed" population—we should listen to what they have to say. Are the results at all reflective of the behavior and attitudes of players in the NFL? We do not know. However, a further question is raised: Did steroid users disproportionately volunteer for the study?

It is believed that estimates of steroid use based on anonymous, self-report surveys underestimate the magnitude of the problem of steroid use in sports[13–16]. Thus one might argue that steroid users were less likely to volunteer for the survey than nonusers and that the steroid users who did volunteer would be proportionally *less* likely to *report* their use in the survey. On the other hand, steroid users were perhaps more likely to volunteer but then deny their use in the survey so as to minimize the public's perception of the problem. It is interesting to note, however, that when the respondents were asked to estimate the level of use among their fellow NFL players, the estimates were quite close to the participants' self-reported level of use (32% other vs. 28% own). Nevertheless, due to the low response rate, the results related to the level of steroid use should *not* be generalized beyond this sample; the findings do, however, make a compelling argument for further research. Clearly, a precise knowledge of the level of drug use is an important step in planning and implementing a drug education and testing program. If the magnitude of the anabolic steroid problem in the NFL is being underestimated, the pressure on those involved in effecting a meaningful solution may be similarly lessened.

An equally important question is, Why did so few players elect to participate in a study that was endorsed and in part developed by the NFLPA? To some this inaction might be interpreted as part of the "veil of secrecy" or "conspiracy of silence" that surrounds drug use in sports[7–9, 13–5]. Perhaps an inherent problem with studies of drug use, even those that guarantee individual and team anonymity, is that they are unable to protect the reputation of the sport. The fear of "guilt by association" and its potential to adversely effect the athlete's place in sports history could result in a hesitancy to volunteer, especially in sports that have traditionally been associated with drug use, such as professional football, powerlifting, and bodybuilding[2, 14, 17–18]. In addition, the players' perception that management holds a less than enthusiastic attitude on curtailing steroid use probably did not enhance the response rate. The majority of players in this study believe that the NFL primarily views steroid use as a public problem and that coaches are, at best, indifferent to the players' steroid use.

Another issue that deserves comment is why we gave attention in our analysis to any prior steroid use as opposed to limiting our focus solely to use within the past twelve months. Anabolic steroids are not necessarily "temporary" performance enhancers in that they are capable of providing the athlete with increased muscle mass and strength, some of which can be maintained for a number of years by training alone. One might then argue that once you use anabolic steroids you are never really the same. Consequently, is there an ethical difference between an NFL player who does not currently use steroids but used them in college to gain enough weight to be drafted, and the aging NFL veteran who used steroids during the past year to keep his job?

It is hoped that the results of this study, combined with those of elite powerlifters[14] and adolescent steroid users[10], will put to rest the often-quoted but never well-documented accounts of surveys claiming that the majority of athletes are willing to die in five years to win a gold medal today[19]. Indeed, the large majority of the NFL players questioned wished to see steroid use stopped and were willing to stop if deleterious health effects were demonstrated.

Although our participants believed that the drug testing program currently in place in the NFL will decrease anabolic steroid use, their mistrust of the accuracy and fairness of the 1989 program should be a matter of concern. This skepticism about the efficacy of drug testing, coupled with the reasonably high levels of perceived steroid use among fellow players, could heighten the incentive to use these drugs.

CONCLUSIONS

The readers, like the authors, are left with difficult choices. One can either dismiss all the findings based on the low response rate or view the 120 respondents as a collection of knowledgeable informants who have shared their insider's view of this controversial issue. Regardless, this study should bolster the cry for further research and help focus its direction. Given that NFL players are role models for thousands of high school and college athletes, the questions raised here are too important to be left unanswered.

REFERENCES

1. Gilbert B: Drugs in Sport: Part 1. Problems in a Turned-On World. Part 2. Something Extra on the Ball. Part 3. High Time to Make Some Rules. *Sports Illustrated*, June 23, June 30, July 7, 1969.

2. Wade N: Anabolic Steroids: Doctors Denounce Them, but Athletes Aren't Listening. *Science* 176: (1972) 1399–1403

3. Lieber J: Steroids: A Problem of Huge Dimensions. *Sports Illustrated*, May 13, 1985.

4. Zimmerman, P: The Agony Must End. *Sports Illustrated*, November 10, 1986.

5. Committee on the Judiciary, United States Senate: Steroids in Amateur and Professional Sports—The Medical and Social Costs of Steroid Abuse. One Hundred First Congress, First Session, April 3, 1989—Newark, DE; May 9, 1989—Washington, D.C.

6. Yesalis C, Anderson W, Buckley W, et al.: Incidence of the Non-Medical Use of Anabolic-Androgenic Steroids. In: Lin, G., and Erinoff, R. eds., *Anabolic Steroid Abuse* (NIDA Research Monograph, 102). National Institute on Drug Abuse: Rockville, MD, 1990.

7. Voy R: *Drugs, Sport, and Politics.* Champaign, IL: Leisure Press, 1990.

8. Dubin, C: *Commission of Inquiry into the use of Drugs and Banned Practices Intended to Increase Athletic Performance.* Canadian Government Publishing Center. Catalogue No. CP32-56/1990E, ISBN 0-660-13610-4, 1990.

9. Francis C: *Speed Trap*. New York: St. Martin's Press, 1990.

10. Buckley WE, Yesalis CE, Friedl KE, et al.: Estimated Prevalence of Anabolic Steroid Use Among Male High School Seniors. *Journal of the American Medical Association*, 260 (23) (1988): 3441–3445.

11. Anderson, W, McKeag D: *The Substance Use and Abuse Habits of College Student-Athletes* (Research Paper #2). Mission, KS: National Collegiate Athletic Association, 1985.

12. Anderson W, Albrecht R, McKeag D, Hough D, McGrew C: Alcohol and Drug Use by Collegiate Athletes. *Physician Sportsmed* 19 (2) (1991): 91–104.

13. Yesalis C, Buckley W, Anderson W, Wang M, Norwig J, Ott O, Puffer J, Strauss R: Athletes' Projections of Anabolic Steroid Use. *Journal of Clinical Sports Medicine*, in press.

14. Yesalis C, Herrick RT, Buckley WE, Friedl KE, Brannon D, Wright JE, Self-Reported use of Anabolic-Androgenic Steroids by Elite Power Lifters. *Physician Sportsmed* 16 (1988): 91–100.

15. Pope H, Katz D, Champoux R: Anabolic-Androgenic Steroid Use Among 1,010 College Men. *Physician Sportsmed* 16 (1988), 75–81.

16. Pope H, Katz D: Affective and Psychotic Symptoms Associated with Anabolic Steroid Use. *American Journal of Psychiatry* 145 (1988): 487–490.

17. Wright J: *Anabolic Steroids and Sports*. Natick, MA: Sports Science Consultants, 1978.

18. Wadler G, Mainline B: *Drugs and the Athlete*. Philadelphia: F.A. Davis Company, 1989.

19. Goldman B: *Death in the Locker Room*. South Bend, IN: Icarus Press, 1984.

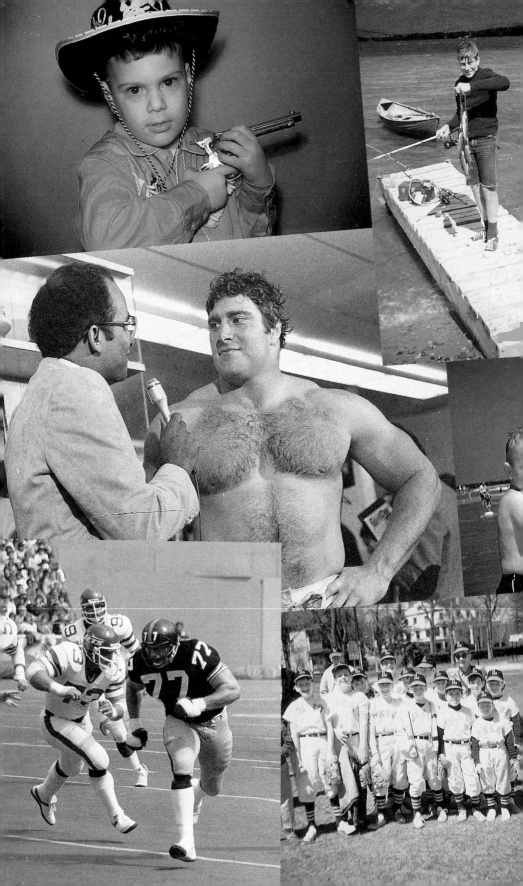